MAMA KNOWS
BREAST

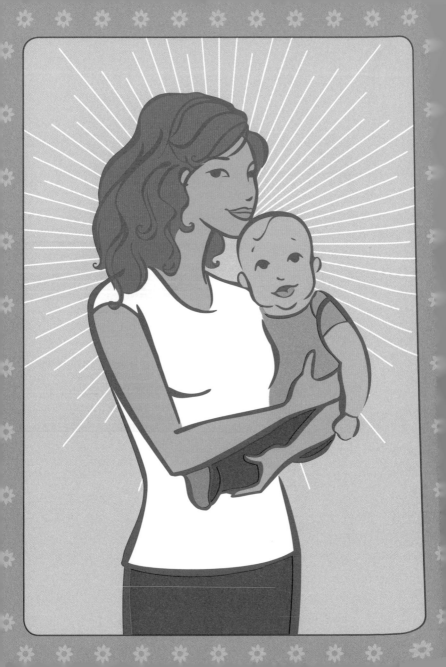

MAMA KNOWS BREAST

a BEGINNER'S GUIDE to *Breastfeeding*

BY ANDI SILVERMAN

QUIRK BOOKS
PHILADELPHIA

Library of Congress Cataloging in Publication Number: 2007925763

ISBN: 978-1-59474-165-4

Printed in China

Typeset in Belizio, Gotham, and Wessex

Designed by Becky Berkheimer

Illustrations by Cindy Luu

Edited by Melissa Wagner

Production management by Chris Veneziale

Distributed in North America by Chronicle Books
680 Second Street
San Francisco, CA 94107

10 9 8 7 6 5 4 3 2 1

Quirk Books
215 Church Street
Philadelphia, PA 19106
www.quirkbooks.com

Disclaimer: This book is not meant to take the place of advice from a qualified medical professional.

Contents

To my husband and sons who made this possible. *Truly.*

WORDS OF WISDOM FROM A PEDIATRICIAN MOM

As a pediatrician, I've seen a lot of babies breastfeed. But it wasn't until I breastfed my own kids—four of them to be exact—that I really learned the ropes.

Each baby was different. One of my children preferred to eat from the "right" side. Another only liked to eat without clothes on. I got pregnant while still breastfeeding one baby. And when the older kids saw me taking care of the newborn, they tried to breastfeed their dolls and "pump" their belly buttons. They also liked to watch me pump, placing bets on which side would produce more milk. "I think that side is winning, mommy!" It's been a few years since I weaned my youngest, but for some reason I still keep my breast pump in my office.

Although your experience will be unique, like everyone, you'll have days when breastfeeding will seem easy and days when it will seem downright impossible. You'll have question after question: Is my baby eating enough? Is he eating too much? Why won't my baby fall asleep unless he's breastfeeding? How do I pump enough milk before going back to work? What's the best way to wean my baby? Can dad do *anything* to help?!

Everyone will give you conflicting advice. Friends and family members mean well, but they don't always have the right answer. Doctors and lactation consultants all have their own perspectives. Books and Web sites have a lot to say—sometimes so much that it can be overwhelming. Knowing whose advice to follow can seem confusing.

The key to success is trying different methods until you find what works for you. Have a sense of humor about it, and don't give up. Most important, always ask for help. That's what we professionals are here for. You may feel alone at times, but rest assured you aren't.

If you aren't ready to pick up the phone just yet, *Mama Knows Breast* is a good first stop. Dads, grandparents, and babysitters will also find some helpful baby advice here. Laughter does lighten the load, and this book will make it all seem much more manageable.

Stephanie Freilich, M.D.
Fellow of the American Academy of Pediatrics
Mount Sinai School of Medicine, New York

THE BREAST OF TIMES, THE WORST OF TIMES

Breasts are everywhere. You just can't escape them. They're all over billboards and magazines, movies and television shows. We worship the cleavage. In fact, it seems like everyone is on "boob watch." Guys are hard-wired to stare, and even women check each other out to see how they "stack up."

Despite all the attention, it's easy to forget that breasts serve a real purpose. It's rare to see people breastfeed, either in public or at home—it's just not part of our culture. We tend to equate babies with bottles and overlook that we're mammals. Mammals, of course, breastfeed to keep their kids alive.

At least that's how it was for me. Before I got pregnant, I really thought of my breasts in only one way. They were kind of cute (if I do say so myself). Even when I was well into my first trimester, I didn't dwell on why they had suddenly morphed from an A to a B to a C. Breastfeeding really wasn't on my radar. I was more worried about the baby's growth.

Breastfeeding was perhaps the one thing I *didn't* worry about when I was pregnant. My mom had breastfed, so I would, too. I naively assumed it would be straightforward. It's what nature intended, so how hard could it be, right? Nevertheless, on the off chance that I might need some guidance, my husband and I attended a breastfeeding class. I even took notes. I had a couple parenting books, too, so I thought I was all set.

When our son was born, I did remember to do a few things I had learned in the class: I fed him as soon as possible after the delivery; he stayed in my recovery room; and I even put a note on his bassinet telling the nurses not to give him a bottle or pacifier. But beyond that, it quickly became clear that I had no idea what I was doing.

As I held the baby to my breast, I couldn't tell if anything was actually happening. Was he eating or just sucking? I tried to ask a nurse, but she was in and out of the room so quickly she barely looked at us. Wanting a little more reassurance, I asked her if a lactation consultant could stop by. Her response was underwhelming—she said that first I had to attend a breastfeeding class. Like a good trooper, I waddled down the hall and then promptly fell asleep in class. So much for my continuing breastfeeding education.

Somehow I muddled through those days in the hospital. But once we were home, I was in for a shock. My breasts, which I had considered big during pregnancy, reached truly gargantuan proportions. My husband even

took to calling me "Torpedo Tits." (Thanks, honey.)
In truth, my girls did look like heat-seeking missiles.
They were so hot and swollen, I stood in the shower
weeping in utter disbelief. Was something wrong with
me? I know I called someone (my doctor? a hospital
nurse? a lactation consultant?), but it's all a blur now.
Eventually, I got some relief by pumping and making
the baby eat more frequently to relieve the pressure.

Those early weeks were the breast of times and
the worst of times. Our son was eating easily and
growing bigger by the day. When he cried, I provided
instant gratification. There were moments of sheer
bliss. But there were also times when breastfeeding
sucked—literally. If I forgot to put pads inside my bra,
I leaked through my clothes. Worst of all, I was exhausted.
Of course I knew that babies didn't sleep much, but
I must not have been paying attention during that
part of breastfeeding class when the teacher said that
newborns eat *every two to three hours, around the clock*.
None of my friends or family had warned me. How
could they have kept this a secret?!

As the months went by, breastfeeding did get easier.
Along the way, I became increasingly bold about where
I breastfed. I did it while dining in a restaurant, shopping

for clothes, and even getting a pedicure. I wasn't an exhibitionist, but if the baby was hungry while I was running an errand, then I stopped to feed him. I was as discreet as possible, but, quite honestly, I wasn't focused on whether or not it made other people uncomfortable. I had to get out of the house, and the baby was coming with me. Bottles weren't an option when we were out and about, since he usually clamped his mouth shut with a scowl at the first taste of a plastic nipple.

Challenges aside, breastfeeding was a bonding experience for me and my husband. We even had a comedy routine that went like this: Dad carries baby to mom: "Here's the Titty Lady! The kitchen is open." Baby spits up all over mom and goes right back to eating: "Boy, this kid can boot and rally." Baby passes out from drinking too much: "He's drunk! He's actually milk drunk!"

All that bonding must have been a good thing, because one night we had a little rendezvous. Our baby was only ten months old, but that night his destiny as a big brother was sealed. Yes, we learned the hard way that breastfeeding is not foolproof birth control. You *can* get pregnant while you're breastfeeding. Trust me. It happened to me, and it could happen to you, too.

The day I found out I was pregnant was also the day I decided to start weaning. My boobs ached, and I didn't have the physical energy to feed one child while another was growing inside me. Weaning, however, wasn't exactly easy. At first, my son refused to take a bottle or sippy cup of formula, and I was afraid he would dehydrate. He launched at least five different types of cups across the apartment before finally accepting one. As for me, I got engorged again since my boobs didn't know what to do with all the milk he wasn't drinking. This time, luckily, I knew how to fix the problem.

All told, it took a month for the baby to kick his nursing habit and for me to turn off the faucets. Of course there was the day, more than a week after he finished breastfeeding, when I spontaneously erupted, soaking our sheets and even the mattress pad.

Now I'm on to Baby 2. For the most part, it's been smooth sailing. There have even been glorious days, when he stops sucking, looks up at me, says "Ah bah bah bah," and then goes right back to eating. But we've had our rough spots. He was such a sleepy newborn that I had to wake him up to nurse. And lately, I've breastfed while running after his older brother in the playground. It's not pretty.

I can still remember one of the last times I nursed our older son. I was sitting in a rocking chair, staring at the river and watching the sunrise. I don't know when that final day will come with our second baby, but I think it's soon. Of course, things could change. Maybe he'll be a bit older than I intend. Maybe a bit younger. No matter when it happens, I know I'll look back on this stage with nostalgia.

Finally, this time around I have a few things on my personal weaning list. First, I want a picture of mom and babe. Nothing cheesy. Just a nice image of the two of us snuggled together. Second, since I won't be pregnant this time around, I have a big plan. I'm throwing out my nursing bras and heading to the department store. I can't wait to see what size I'll be.

❖ ❖ ❖

After two babies, I certainly have my share of war stories. But all moms do, whether they breastfeed or bottle feed. Which brings me to an important point—breastfeeding is truly a matter of personal choice. It's up to you. Your life, your decision. Do some reading, get expert advice, and then make up your own mind. Whatever happens, don't despair. Whether you breastfeed for one week, one month, one year, or longer, you'll be the center of your baby's universe.

As for me, I started to write *Mama Knows Breast* when I realized that I knew more about my baby's car seat, stroller, and crib than I did about breastfeeding. So I did my homework and talked to doctors, lactation consultants, and moms. The result is a collection of all the things I wish someone had told me when I was pregnant for the first time.

I wish I had known about the ups and downs of breastfeeding (chapter 1) and how to actually do it (chapters 2 and 3). I *really* wish someone had warned me about the lack of sleep (chapter 4). I was able to muddle my way through breastfeeding in public (chapter 5), and my husband and I managed to figure out how to make breastfeeding a "couple's" activity (chapter 6). But I would have loved honest information about how breastfeeding can affect your sex life (chapter 7), and I really needed some guidance on weaning (chapter 8).

So think of this book as your new best friend. Imagine sitting around a table with your friends and letting it all hang out. What would they say about biting teeth? Stockpiling pumped milk and formula?

Warding off horny husbands? Whatever their advice, they would be there for you. Now *Mama Knows Breast* is here for you, too.

If you're still expecting, start banking your sleep *now*. Put this book down and take a nap or call it a night. If your baby is already born, prop your feet up on your ottoman, latch him onto your breast, and wedge this book under his bottom. Gently turn the page with one hand while supporting his head with the other one. If he's older, be prepared to keep him from ripping the pages apart.

It's Titty Time.

Chapter 1

THE PROS AND CONS OF BREASTFEEDING

Before your baby is even born, your body gears up for the task ahead. Your breasts get bigger and your nipples get darker until they resemble a bull's-eye. It's the perfect target for your newborn, who can't see very far at first and has to feel and smell her way around. Your breasts also start to produce colostrum, an antibody-rich milk. Then, a few days after you give birth, your mature milk will "come in." You may see veins where they've never appeared before, and your breasts, which you probably already thought couldn't get any bigger, may look and feel like they belong to someone else. You might feel a slight tingling sensation when you breastfeed. Of course everyone is different, and some women might not notice or feel any changes at all, even if their milk has arrived.

A little preparation will guide you through the experience. Learning about the ups and downs of breastfeeding before your baby is born may even help you decide how to proceed. As you're contemplating all this, remember that breastfeeding is a highly personal experience. Some women love it, others hate it. How will you feel? No way to know until you give it a try and consider the pros and cons.

The 10 Best Things About Breastfeeding

(1)   Breastfeeding is good for your baby's health. Breast milk is the "gold standard" for babies. It's full of antibodies and nutrients. Research shows that breastfeeding can protect a baby from a range of infectious illnesses and diseases, including diarrhea, ear infections, bacterial meningitis, SIDS, diabetes, obesity, asthma, and some childhood cancers. Some studies also show that breastfed babies perform better on tests of cognitive development.

(2)   Breastfeeding is good for *your* health. After your baby is born, breastfeeding increases the uterine contractions that help your body return to its pre-pregnancy state. Over time, breastfeeding will also help you lose weight because it burns calories. Think about it—you can lose weight by sitting still and feeding your baby. You don't even need your sneakers! Research shows that breastfeeding can also reduce the risk of Type II diabetes, ovarian and breast cancers, and possibly osteoporosis.

(3) **Breastfeeding gives you time to bond with your baby.**
Since you're spending countless hours locked in a warm
embrace, you'll get to know every nook and cranny of
your baby's face and body. You'll recognize the little
clues in her expressions and mannerisms that indicate
whether she's hungry, tired, or ready to burp. Once
you've got that down, you're one step closer to preventing
her from spiraling into full-blown hysterical crying.
Plus, isn't it pretty cool that you can nourish another
human being with your own body?

(4) **You can feed your baby anywhere, anytime.** You're a
veritable moveable feast. You can take your baby out to
a restaurant or on a plane without having to remember
to pack bottles and formula. Have boob, will travel.

(5) **You don't have to prepare a bottle.** When the little
guy is hungry, all you have to say is, "One boob, coming
right up!" and the crying stops. On the other hand,
preparing formula and heating the bottle to the perfect
temperature take time. All the while, your baby is
screaming, "WAITER, I'M HUNGRY!"

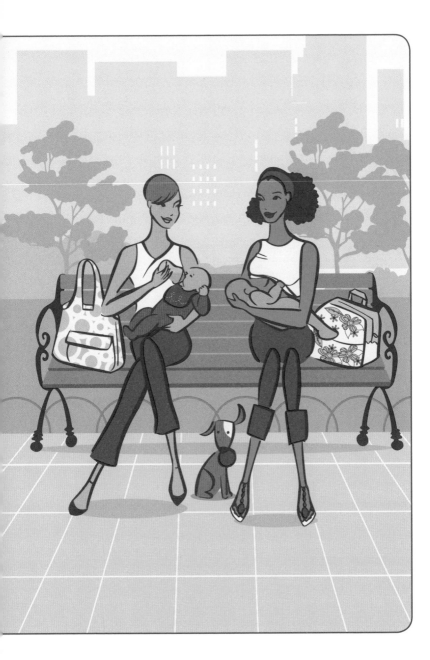

Mama Data

An annual study conducted by the Ross Products Division of Abbott Laboratories (the same company that makes the formula Similac) shows that breastfeeding rates in the United States have increased exponentially during the past thirty years. In 1971, roughly 25 percent of women breastfed their babies at birth; by 2006, 64 percent of women did so. There's also a trend to continue breastfeeding longer. Six months after giving birth, only 5 percent of moms were still breastfeeding in 1971; in 2006, 30 percent of moms continued breastfeeding.

(6) **You don't have to clean or sterilize bottles.** You probably already feel like you don't have a moment to yourself, so who wants to add to the mess piling up in the kitchen sink?

(7) **You might not get your period for a while.**
Breastfeeding can suppress your monthly menstrual cycle. But be careful–breastfeeding is not perfect birth control. If your baby is older, eating solid foods, and you aren't breastfeeding day and night, you could start to ovulate again. You'll need to use condoms or get yourself a prescription for a progesterone-only pill.

(8) Breastfeeding costs a lot less than formula. Although there are expenses involved in breastfeeding—you may need nursing bras, nursing pads, a pump, and a nursing shirt or two—the amount you'll spend doesn't come close to the cost of a year's worth of formula. By some rough estimates, formula can cost as much as $3,000 per year.

(9) Breastfeeding is good for the environment. Since your breast milk comes in a waste-free reusable container, breastfeeding is environmentally friendly. If you use formula, you'll be sending bottles, nipples, and empty formula cans to a landfill. Plus, manufacturing and transporting formula require fuel. Can you say *global warming*?

(10) You still have that big-boobed maternal glow. Breastfeeding will definitely make your breasts bigger. Some women have even reported growing from an A to a D in cupsize! Some folks welcome this change; others don't. Either way, you'll lose some of your new shapeliness when you stop breastfeeding.

The 10 Worst Things About Breastfeeding

(1) **No one else can do your job.** If you are exclusively breastfeeding–in other words, if you're not supplementing with bottles of formula or pumped breast milk–you're always on call. Want to get a haircut? Go out to dinner? Spend a night away from home? These activities can be a challenge unless you can get out of the house and back home between feedings.

(2) **Sleep deprivation.** There is no rest for the weary, especially if your baby doesn't take a bottle so someone else can feed him while you sleep. Newborns eat around the clock, so say goodbye to an uninterrupted night's sleep. After a few months your baby will be able to go longer stretches without waking up. Eventually, he'll be asleep before the sun sets and wake up when it rises.

(3) **The breast pump.** You'll have to make time to pump if you plan to be away from the baby for more than a few hours. And if you don't pump, your breasts will start to hurt, and they may even leak. Plus, if you don't feed or pump, your milk supply will decrease. So, get ready to lug around

From the Mouths of Moms

During my daughter's christening, I stood on the altar feeling every inch the happiest mummy in the world. Then my sister caught my eye. She was gesticulating wildly and pulling at her top. With horror I realized she was trying to get me to pull my jacket closed. I glanced down, and to my utter embarrassment I saw that the front of my lovely new lilac dress was turning a deep purple as my milk leaked everywhere.

— SINEAD, WWW.BREASTFEEDINGMUMS.COM

a heavy breast pump or stash a smaller, hand-powered pump in your purse (see page 59). Then comes the real challenge—finding a private place to pump and a good way to store your milk until you get home.

(4) **You'll have to get used to feeding in public.** Unless you plan on becoming a hermit, you won't always be ensconced in the privacy of your own home each time the baby needs to eat. You'll invariably find yourself in the middle of a department store or the supermarket when it's snack time. Inconvenient? Yes. Potentially embarrassing? Yes. Annoying comments from family,

friends, and strangers? Yes. What's a mom to do?
See chapter 5, "Breastfeeding Etiquette," for pointers.

(**5**)   **Alcohol and caffeine in moderation.** As with everything
mommy related, you'll find conflicting opinions on how
much alcohol and caffeine you can consume. So here's
the bottom line: Alcohol and caffeine can show up in
your milk, so they're okay only in moderation and at
appropriate times. In other words, no coffee if you're about
to feed your baby and then put him to sleep. As for alcohol,
an occasional drink is fine, though excessive drinking
is not good for your baby (see page 71).

(**6**)   **Leakage.** Some women leak breast milk. Sometimes
one breast leaks while the other one is feeding the baby.
Sometimes it happens spontaneously, in the middle
of a romantic dinner. Not everyone faces this problem,
of course. But if you do, you'll need to wear pads
(disposable or washable) inside your bra. Some women
even carry a change of clothes, or at least a sweater,
scarf, or coat, to hide unwelcome splotches.

(7) **Your husband has to share your boobs with someone else.**
Since you started dating, he has had you all to himself.
Now he'll have to adjust to sharing. Let's face it—if the
baby is hungry and crying, your husband will just have
to wait his turn. This might require some adjustments in
your relationship. (See chapter 7, "Sex and Relaxation.")

From the Mouths of Moms

As a second-time mom, and an Ob-Gyn to boot, I didn't anticipate having
trouble nursing our new baby. But after an unexpected C-section and a
stay in the newborn intensive care unit, Joey would not nurse. I also had
a milk supply problem. I spent the first two weeks of his life pumping
around the clock to build up my milk supply from practically nothing.
After about six weeks he finally learned to latch on, and I was able to stop
giving him bottles of formula. There were so many times I nearly gave
up because of fatigue and frustration, but it was so worth the effort.

— DAWN, NEW HAVEN, CONNECTICUT

(8) **Your husband can feel left out of the baby-bonding process.**
If you're doing all the feeding and not supplementing
with bottles of formula or pumped breast milk, your
husband might feel like he's missing something special.
If so, he can still take care of the burping, diapering,
bathing, clothing, swaddling, cuddling, reading, strolling,
and playing. Guaranteed, he'll feel better! (See chapter 6,
"How Your Spouse Can Help.")

(9) **Discomfort.** If your baby is latched on well, breastfeeding
shouldn't hurt. But for some, there's no getting around a
bit of discomfort. Somewhere along the way, something
is bound to feel less than optimal. Maybe it's engorgement,
a blister, or bite from an itty-bitty baby tooth. Rest assured,
however, that most problems are fixable; just get help as
soon as possible. (See chapter 2, "Operating Instructions.")

(10) **YOU WILL NEED HELP!!** Nature intended us to
breastfeed, but breastfeeding is far from "second nature."
It takes practice. Watch another woman breastfeed, get
pointers, and don't be shy about asking for help. Although
your friends and family might have good tips, it's often
better to get the advice of a professional—a lactation
consultant (see page 99).

Formula Facts

In the mid-nineteenth century, chemists began concocting different "formulas." These mixtures contained ingredients such as cow's milk, wheat, sugar, and water. Companies marketed these varying formulas to women and doctors as a nutritious way to feed babies, and by the twentieth century, women regularly used formula. So what exactly is formula? Basically, it's a substitute for human breast milk. Scientists don't know the precise composition of breast milk, but they've tried to get as close as possible.

In some developing countries, breastfeeding is safer for infants than formula-feeding. In developed countries, however, where women have access to clean water, formula-feeding is considered a viable alternative to breastfeeding. In the United States, the U.S. Food and Drug Administration (FDA) regulates the composition of formula. There are strict guidelines about what ingredients have to be in formula—certain vitamins, minerals, protein, and fats. But take a walk down the baby aisle in your supermarket or drugstore, and you're bound to find the choice of formulas overwhelming.

There are soy-based formulas and milk-based formulas. Some are powders. Some are ready to pour. How do you choose? If you think you want formula, your safest bet is to get your pediatrician's advice. Once your baby is twelve months old, with a doctor's approval, you can switch from formula to cow's milk.

It's Your Choice

People are nosy. For months they've had probing questions: When are you due? Is it a boy or a girl? Do you have a name yet? Once the baby is born, there's a new set of questions: Are you breastfeeding? Does the baby take a bottle? Have you tried formula? Even worse, everyone seems to have an opinion about how long you should breastfeed. If you stop after one month, you might hear, "Breast is best. Maybe you should go longer." If you're still breastfeeding at one year, you might hear, "When are you going to stop?" All this prying can get downright annoying.

If so, don't feel bad about suggesting, ever so politely, that people back off. You're the only one who has to feed your baby, and you'll choose what works best for you. You'll feel enough guilt about all the other things you are—or aren't—doing for her, so try to eliminate one more pressure you put on yourself.

Most important, don't feel like you have to stick to your pre-birth game plan. When you were pregnant, you may have felt certain that you would breastfeed, but then once the baby arrived you decided it wasn't for you. Or maybe you were convinced you would use formula but found instead that you preferred to breastfeed. Whatever the case, there's no shame in changing your mind. You can't know how you'll feel, or what will happen, until that baby pops out.

From the Mouths of Moms

When I told my mother I was going to breastfeed, she responded, "Why would you want to do that to yourself?" She said she never even considered breastfeeding when I was born in 1967. She told me the nurses just assumed she'd want ice packs to stop her milk from coming in painfully. I tried to explain to her that it wasn't about me; it was about what was best for the baby. I went over all the benefits and how it is really encouraged now, but she still can't believe I plan on breastfeeding for more than a few weeks.

— SAM, BURLINGTON, VERMONT

No matter what you decide, do yourself a big favor—buy at least one nursing bra to bring to the hospital. You won't have time to leisurely shop for bras when you get home. Just do the best you can to figure out your bra size. Then, sit back and enjoy the roller-coaster ride.

Chapter 2

OPERATING
INSTRUCTIONS

Remember what it was like to learn to drive?
An automatic car was hard, and a stick shift was even
harder. Breastfeeding falls somewhere in between.
It's tricky, but not impossible. You'll get the hang of it,
with practice—sometimes weeks and weeks of practice.
Ideally, you'll want to give it a go for the first time as
soon as possible after you deliver the baby, preferably
within the hour. Over the next weeks, you're bound
to have a few false starts and stops. So here's a basic
tip: If you have a problem, find a reliable instructor as
quickly as possible. No need to play tough guy. Talk to
a lactation consultant, doctor, nurse, midwife, doula,
or friend. Check out an online community or find a
support group at your hospital. You can also contact
the local chapter of La Leche League, the international
group that has been promoting breastfeeding for more
than fifty years (see page 99). In the meantime, here
are some guidelines that may help make things easier.
Ladies, start your engines.

Holding Your Baby

Put yourself in your baby's position for a second. What's she thinking about? Some basic stuff. She wants to eat, breathe, and feel safely held in your arms. So it's your job, mama, to put your baby at ease while she's eating. There are different ways to comfortably hold her, and soon enough you'll figure out what feels best. Here are some options to test drive.

(1) **Cradle Hold.** This is the classic. Your baby's head rests on your forearm, his stomach is against yours, and his ears, shoulders, and hips should be in a straight line. Keep his inside arm by his side. If necessary, use your free hand to hold your breast. Try using a pillow to raise the baby to the level of your breast. This position works well as you become more experienced and your baby gets older and sprawls across your lap; but just after birth, you might have an easier time with one of the next three holds.

(2) **Cross-Cradle Hold.** This is the best hold to try with a newborn, and especially a premature baby. The baby is in the same position as in the Cradle Hold, but this time you hold him with the opposite arm. Put the palm of your hand between his shoulder blades; your thumb and fingers go just below his ears.

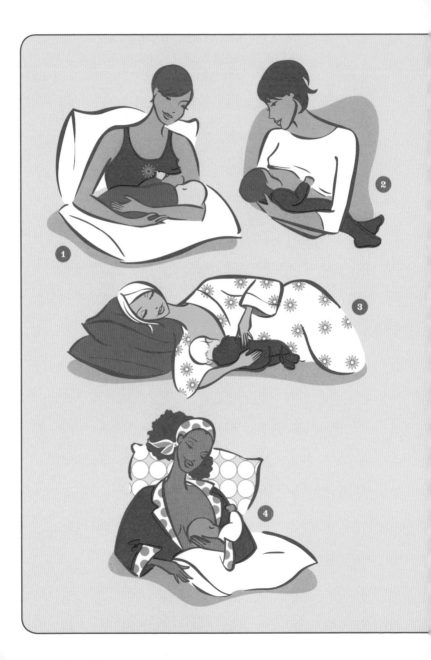

(3)   **Side-Lying Hold.** Lie on your side with the baby facing
you. You might want to support his head in the crook
of your arm to keep his mouth level with your nipple.
This position is tricky and can make you feel like a
contortionist at times, but it's great if you're really tired.
Just keep a good grip on the baby in case you fall asleep.

(4)   **Football Hold.** Hold the baby along your side, supporting
his back with your forearm and resting his head and neck
in your hand. This position is quite effective if you've had a
C-section because it avoids putting pressure on your stomach.
It's also good for feeding twins at the same time. And for all
babies, it can help you keep an eye on the baby's mouth.

From the Mouths of Moms

The first night in the hospital, I lay there and propped Sophie up on her
side. But I had nowhere to put my bottom arm, and her latch would fail.
Later I saw a picture of a woman, semi-reclined, with her son cradled
in the *crook of her elbo*w. I couldn't believe I hadn't realized what to do
with that arm. Now Sophie nurses beautifully.

— ELLEN, TAVERNIER, FLORIDA

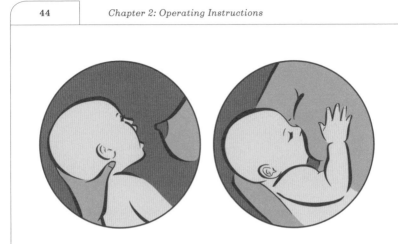

The Latch

By now you've probably accepted that it's your job to teach your
kid a thing or two for at least the next twenty years. Though
math lessons and safe-sex talks are still years down the road,
at this early stage you can focus on something a little more
basic—teaching your baby how to suck, or latch on to, your
breast. Your baby does have a "rooting reflex" that causes her to
make sucking motions and turn towards your breast, but she
needs to learn what to do once she gets there. Of course you're
learning this trick, too, so it's sort of the blind leading the
blind. If something doesn't feel right, stop and start over again.
Eventually you'll be able to latch her on without even thinking
about what you're doing.

(1) **Open Up.** Hold the baby's chest and chin against your breast, causing her to tilt her head back and open her mouth. It will look like your nipple is going up her nose. If she hasn't opened her mouth on her own, touch your nipple to her top lip.

(2) **Make contact.** The objective is to get her mouth to completely cover your nipple *and* as much of your areola, the dark ring around your nipple, as possible. Once her mouth is open wide, quickly push one hand against her shoulder blades to bring her onto your breast, chin first. Make sure you bring the baby to your breast, not your breast to the baby. Try not to bend your wrist or her head. You can hold your breast with your other hand; think of the letter "C"–your thumb goes on top of your breast and your other fingers support it from underneath. The baby's chin and cheeks should touch your breast and her nose should be clear. If all is working well, the latch shouldn't hurt. With both of her lips rolled open in the proper position, she'll look like a fish taking a big gulp!

(3) **Dinner is served.** Try feeding your baby "on demand."
In other words, feed him when he tells you he's hungry by
crying, rooting, licking his lips, or sucking his fist. There
are several ways to determine if your baby is getting milk.

- The baby is swallowing, not just sucking. Sucking is
  quick and shallow, whereas swallowing is deep and
  rhythmic (about one swallow per second). You might see
  the baby's chin move open, pause, and then close. You
  might also hear the baby make a throaty bullfrog-like
  noise. Sometimes, however, the swallowing is silent.
- Your breasts feel softer after a feeding.
- You see milk in the baby's mouth.
- The baby no longer "roots" for food.
- You may feel your milk "letting down." This can
  be a tingling sensation in your breasts. Not everyone
  experiences this, especially in the beginning.

(4) **Letting go.** Your baby may decide that she's had enough,
and she'll let go of your breast all by herself. Sometimes
you'll have to help her. If you want to switch to the other
breast, or redo the latch because it's uncomfortable, put
your finger in the corner of the baby's mouth and gently
pull back toward her ear to break the suction. She'll let
you go without doing much damage to your nipple.

From the Mouths of Moms

One night while nursing I looked down and the baby's mouth was covered in blood—my vampire child. There was a small cut on my breast that one of the twins had sucked open. Nice. It was amusing to a certain extent, because I sometimes felt like they were little animals suckling me to death.

— ANOUK, LOS ANGELES, CALIFORNIA

(5) Switching Sides. It's important to nurse evenly from each breast to stimulate milk production and prevent engorgement. Try to start each feeding on a different side, and switch sides during each feeding. There are no rules about how long to nurse on each side. Simply switch when the baby's swallowing slows down or you feel the need to empty the other breast.

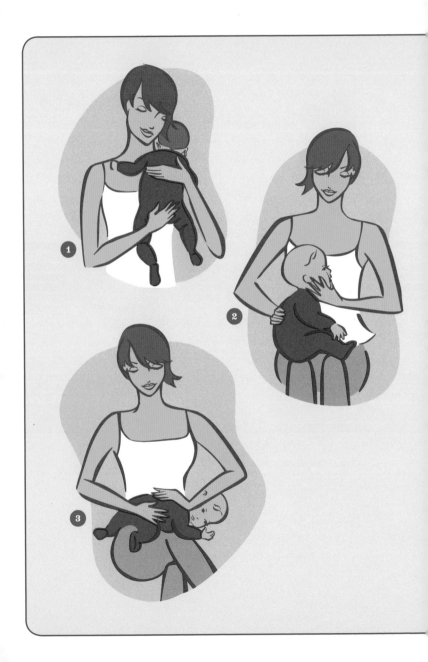

Burping

In general, you probably consider burping to be rather uncouth. Now, however, you'll hang on your baby's every belch as if it were a message from the Oracle at Delphi.

When your baby burps, you'll know he has relieved the pressure in his stomach from air he may have swallowed while eating. You can try to burp him after he's finished with one breast and before he starts the other. Remember, every kid is different. Some never need to burp, whereas others do it all the time. Here are some techniques for getting the kid to let one rip.

(1)   **The Over-the-Shoulder Hold:** Hold the baby under his tushy so that his head rests on your shoulder. Use your free hand to pat and rub his middle to lower back.

(2)   **Sitting Upright on Your Lap:** Sit the baby sideways, supporting his chin with one hand. Let him lean forward to put pressure on his stomach. Rub his back with your free hand.

(3)   **Stomach Down:** Lay the baby across your lap with his head facing sideways. Raise his head slightly by crossing your legs. Put one hand on his tushy and rub his back with your other hand.

Troubleshooting

Gas can make your baby squirm, grimace, and even scream
in agony. If you can't get the baby to reward your efforts with
the satisfying sound of a belch, try placing him on his back
and gently pushing his knees toward his chest. He just might
pass a little gas from the other end!

Spitting Up

While we're on the topic of burping, don't forget that babies also
tend to spit up a fair amount. Whether your baby is breastfeeding
or drinking formula, he can leave a nice little deposit that may
land on your shoulder, roll down your back, or hit the floor with a
resounding splat. So don't forget to wear a burp cloth. And, tacky
though it may sound, consider a slipcover for your fancy couch.

Is He Eating Enough?

With gravity, what goes up must come down. With breastfeeding,
what goes in must come out. In other words, if your baby is
peeing and pooping, then you know he's getting something
to eat. Keeping a journal of feedings and diaper changes will
help you focus on this.

Newborns eat eight to twelve times a day, that is, every two to three hours. They can poop three to four times and pee five to eight times each day. If you have a particularly sleepy baby, you'll have to wake him up to make sure he eats regularly.

After about a month, feedings become less frequent. Every three to four hours is sufficient. The number of poops may decrease when the baby is more than a month old. Even one poop a week is not unheard of!

The chief indication that your baby is well-fed is that he is gaining weight. Most babies lose some weight the first few days after birth, but they'll soon gain it back. Your pediatrician will record the baby's stats so that you know he is on the right track.

Double Trouble: Feeding More Than One Baby

Everywhere you look, you see parents struggling to push double strollers down the street. Whether it's because of twins or just two kids who are close in age, many moms are faced with the possibility of breastfeeding more than one child at a time. The emotional and physical logistics can seem daunting. How can there possibly be enough of mom to go around? As you consider how to handle the situation, remember that the amount of milk you have is based on supply and demand. The more your babies suck and swallow, the more milk you'll make.

From the Mouths of Moms

I don't know how women who exclusively breastfeed twins do it. When our twins were really little, I'd get one latched on, go for the second, and the first would "fall" off my breast. So I'd get the first back on and the second would roll off. I resorted to breastfeeding and bottle-feeding at the same time. I sat on the floor using my knees to support one baby while the other one sat in a bouncy seat. I did this for four months and then had to stop because my milk supply just couldn't keep up.

— ANNE, NEWTON, MASSACHUSETTS

Nursing Twins

Got twins? Forget about doing anything other than feeding and diapering for the first few weeks with your newborns. Line up someone else to cook and do your laundry. Don't plan on checking e-mails or keeping up with things at work. Once your multiples arrive, you're in for the long haul.

In the beginning, try nursing the babies one at a time so that you can really concentrate on getting a proper "latch" with each baby. Once all three of you have it figured out, you can nurse both babies at once. It certainly will save you time! Each baby can eat one side at each feeding, but alternate the sides every time. If that's too hard to remember, try switching every twenty-four hours.

Since breastfeeding twins is definitely double trouble, and certainly not for everyone, some moms supplement breast milk with formula. If you don't want to supplement, make sure you establish a good milk supply early on by either feeding frequently or pumping if your babies have to be in the NICU because they were born early.

Tandem Nursing a Toddler and a Newborn

If you *merely* have two babies close in age, you have it a little easier than juggling twins or triplets—but not much. You're faced with the challenge of balancing the needs of an utterly helpless newborn with your slightly more independent toddler. Some women will wean the older baby as soon as they become pregnant. Others will nurse all through pregnancy and then tandem nurse or breastfeed both children at the same time.

Like any parenting dilemma, the decision can be both emotional and practical. Your newborn and your toddler need your attention, and tandem feeding is certainly one way to take care of that. But it's not the only option. Ultimately, the choice is a personal one. If you choose to give tandem nursing a try, always feed the newborn first to make sure her needs are satisfied. If you're feeling overwhelmed, try limiting the times the older one nurses.

Even if you've already weaned your older child, you can never be sure of how he will react to seeing the newborn nurse. What if he asks if he can breastfeed again? What should you do? If you tell him no, he may do anything from nod in agreement to throw a screaming tantrum. Say yes, and he may just walk away, comforted to know that the milk bar is still open. Then again, he could take you up on your offer.

Maintenance Tips

When you're on an airplane, the flight attendant's usual preflight safety spiel goes something like this: "If the aircraft should experience a sudden loss of pressure, oxygen masks will drop from the overhead compartment. If you are traveling with small children, put on your own mask before helping others." The same principle applies to taking care of your baby. There's no way you can help her if you've passed out—albeit from hunger, exhaustion, or illness. In other words, you need to take care of yourself in order to take care of her. Here's how to achieve optimal working condition for your boobs.

From the Mouths of Moms

While I nursed our newborn, my older son often came to watch. He'd kiss my breasts, or pat them and say, "Mommy, I love your breasts!" My husband knew the breastfeeding had made an impression when he walked into our son's room one day and saw him holding his stuffed animal to his nipple, offering milk!

— LINDA, WASHINGTON, D.C.

✿ *Aim for the milk supply trifecta: food, drink, and sleep.*
You may have heard it before, but it bears repeating—sleep when the baby sleeps. Yes, that's right; you get a sanctioned nap in the middle of the day! As for food, eat a well-balanced diet and drink enough water to prevent dehydration.

✿ *Avoid underwire bras and bras that are too small.*
Wearing a supportive bra is important for comfort, but bras that either are too tight or have underwires can block your milk ducts.

✿ *Don't suffer in silence.* If you're having a problem, get help and get help fast. You don't have to be a hero and tough things out. No one's handing out a martyr medal here. Here's a list of common problems and suggested solutions.

Flat or inverted nipples: If your nipples are flat or inverted, your baby may have trouble latching on. A lactation consultant can show you how to use your fingers or a pump to draw out your nipples. A nipple shield can help the baby latch on (see page 79).

Sore nipples: Soreness can range from mild to severe. You can even have cracks that bleed. Try to improve the baby's latch, rub breast milk or a lanolin cream on your breasts, and pump, instead of nursing, until you heal.

Engorgement: When you first start breastfeeding a newborn, or when you miss a feeding, your breasts may become engorged. Your boobs will feel swollen, hot, and painful. Your nipples may even look extended. To solve this problem, get the milk out! Feed the baby or pump. Use warm compresses for just a few minutes to get the milk flowing. After nursing or pumping, ice packs can relieve the pain. Gently massaging the breast is helpful, too. For extreme engorgement, here's a tried-and-true home remedy—cabbage leaves! Wash a leaf and put it directly on your breast. Leave it on for fifteen to twenty minutes, three times per day. Don't use cabbage longer than that because it can affect milk supply. Always check with your doctor before taking any pain medication.

From the Mouths of Moms

With my first baby, I had cracks the size of the Grand Canyon! Open
wounds. I had three weeks of the worst pain I've ever felt before I figured out what was wrong. And it took seven people to crack my case!
I spoke to three midwives, a visiting nurse, two friends, and a lactation
consultant. Finally, it was the lactation consultant who suggested using
Neosporin after each feeding and to nurse on only one breast for each
feeding, letting the other heal. She also showed me how to get the baby
to latch on properly. It was another three weeks before I was healed.
With my second child, I went straight to the same lactation consultant
as soon as I got home from the hospital.

— JEN, HERMOSA BEACH, CALIFORNIA

Plugged Duct: A mildly tender lump could be a plugged
duct. You might even see a white spot on your nipple.
To get the milk flowing again, frequently feed your baby
and massage your breast. Warm compresses just before
feeding or pumping help, too. If the lump doesn't go away
after feedings, see your doctor as soon as possible to make
sure the lump isn't something more serious, such as breast
cancer (see page 81).

Mastitis: If you have a fever, flulike symptoms, and painful lumps or redness in your breasts, you may have mastitis. This can happen because of engorgement, plugged ducts, or cracked or bleeding nipples. Your doctor may prescribe an antibiotic to help fight the infection. You'll also need to get a lot of rest and frequently feed the baby from the side that hurts (see page 80).

Yeast Infection or Thrush: Soreness, burning, and itching can be signs of a yeast infection on your nipples. Your doctor may give you an antifungal cream. Your baby may have an infection in his mouth or diaper area as well, so he might need treatment, too.

From the Mouths of Moms

I nursed Charlie for seven weeks without incident, but then one day the "red dot" appeared—a tiny red bump on my right nipple. It looked harmless, but I howled with pain when Charlie latched on. My obstetrician suggested that I apply lanolin and contact a lactation consultant. About a week later, the dot disappeared as suddenly as it had arrived.

— JILL, JACKSONVILLE, FLORIDA

Pumping

Like breastfeeding, pumping is highly individual. It's easy for some women and impossible for others. Some folks have a love affair with their pump since it enables them to give their baby breast milk in absentia. Others think their pump is an electric torture device that makes them feel like a cow. Bottom line, if breastfeeding, you're bound to have to deal with a pump at some point. Here are some basic pumping tips.

Choosing and Caring for a Pump

Both mechanical and hand-powered devices are available. Hand-powered pumps are less expensive and are small enough to fit inside your purse (provided your bag isn't a dainty little clutch). On the downside, manual pumps are slow and tiring for your hand. Mechanical pumps are the way to go if you have to pump multiple times a day, and you want to get it done as quickly as possible. Some hospitals rent mechanical pumps. It's also worth investigating whether your insurance will cover the cost of your pump.

Experts offer differing opinions on how best to wash or sterilize your pump. Some advise using boiling water to clean the pieces, whereas others recommend soap and water. Your safest bet is to follow the manufacturer's directions for your model.

Storing and Thawing Milk

Freshly pumped milk is safe for your baby for roughly six hours at room temperature or eight days in the refrigerator. You can also freeze breast milk for as long as six months. To defrost frozen milk, leave it in the fridge (up to 24 hours only) or hold the container under running water—no microwaving or stove-top boiling. Only use plastic bags specifically designed for storing milk.

Pumping Tips

✿ *The more you pump, the more milk you'll have.*
   Breastfeeding follows the simple economic principle of supply and demand. Pump or feed your baby more, and you'll have more milk. Pump or feed less, and you'll make less milk. To increase your supply, pump at the same time every day. Once your milk has stopped flowing, pump for two more minutes— the more stimulation, the better.

✿ *Pump between your morning feedings.* Your milk supply is most plentiful in the morning. Take advantage of that phenomenon by pumping in the morning.

✿ *If you're away from your baby, pump at the same times that your baby would be eating.* That will allow you to keep your milk supply at the right level for your baby's needs.

From the Mouths of Moms

I pumped whenever I could. Even in the car. If people can talk on their cell phones while driving, why can't I pump? Anyway, when my baby was about seven weeks old, we went to visit my parents for about five days. When I came home, I noticed that the freezer door was ajar. It wasn't wide open, but open enough so that the cold air was escaping. Each of the more than 100 bags of milk I'd stored had melted—there wasn't one left that was still frozen. I called my pediatrician, who told me that I couldn't use them. I begged and pleaded and said that they were still cold, but she insisted that I throw them away. I was distraught. I had lost 100 bags of liquid gold and I had to go back to work! I eventually built my supply back up, but I refused to throw the "bad milk" away. I think the baby was ten months old when I finally dumped it. I literally cried as I opened each bag and watched the milk go down the drain.

— TESSA, COLUMBIA, SOUTH CAROLINA

✿ **Loosen up.** You'll need to relax to get your milk flowing. Try looking at a picture of your little cherub, smelling an item of her clothing, or listening to a recording of her baby babble.

✿ **A watched pot never boils.** Don't look at the collection bottles while you're pumping. The first few times you pump, you may not get much of anything. It will feel like it's taking forever just to get one ounce out of your boob. Also, your pump will never extract as much as your baby can. Babies are perfectly designed little inventions. Pumps, try as they may, just don't come close.

✿ **If you have to pump at work, don't be afraid to tell your boss.** Some states have laws requiring employers to provide appropriate nursing rooms for employees. For more advice on pumping at work, see page 103.

From the Mouths of Moms

I had a very easy time nursing, but a miserable time pumping. I recorded an audiotape of our baby crying when she was hungry and played it when I pumped. Something about the sound of her crying let my body know to release the milk.

— LAURA, BOSTON, MASSACHUSETTS

✿ ***Multitask with a pumping bra.*** There are bras specifically designed to hold the cups of your breast pump in place. Just hook yourself up, turn on the machine, and pump, hands free. You can talk on the phone, send e-mails, read the newspaper, or address envelopes for your baby announcements.

Déjà Poo

After talking so much about milk, we have to consider what happens to that milk. It's a little crass to mention it, but there's just no way around dealing with dirty diapers. You're going to have to get used to pee in your hair, poop under your fingernails, and the joys of the public-restroom changing table.

Likewise, you'll soon learn to factor the time it takes to change diapers into your daily routine. Be prepared for the déjà-poo cycle: It's inevitable that once you've changed the baby's diaper; dressed her in her snowsuit, hat, and mittens; and strapped her into her stroller, she will ever so politely leave a little deposit in her pants, and the changing process will have to start all over again. Here are some tried-and-true diapering directions.

✿ ***Repack your diaper bag every night.*** Never, ever, ever forget to pack a diaper bag. If you repack your bag at the end of each day, you're less likely to leave home without all the items you might need. Stuff that bag as full as possible!

❀ ***Buy diapers, wipes, and laundry detergent in bulk.***
"Emergency preparedness" is your mantra. Buy as if a hurricane was about to hit and you're going to be stuck indoors for the next week.

❀ ***Make your own wipes.*** You can use cotton squares soaked in water instead of packaged wipes. Paper towels are another option.

❀ ***Consider buying a diaper trash can.*** These newfangled contraptions, complete with special bag inserts, really do wonders for containing the stink.

❀ ***Use supermarket plastic bags to hold dirty diapers.***
If you don't have a specially designed diaper trash can, you can always use supermarket plastic bags to hold each dirty diaper. These are especially useful for diaper changes when you're away from home. After all, it's not polite to leave an odorous trail in your friend's apartment.

❀ ***Use a "tushy pad" during diaper changes.*** A "tushy pad" is any old material placed under the baby's bottom to minimize the mess. As you'd expect, there are pads specifically designed with this in mind; they have a rubbery backing to contain leaks. You can also use the blue pads found in surgical supply stores and pet stores. If all else fails, paper towels will do the trick.

From the Mouths of Moms

After our baby was born, I was desperate to find a hands-free pumping bra. But the one store in town that carried them said it would take a week to get one. So I did what any warm-blooded Alaskan would do—I jury-rigged my own system. I took an old tube top that hadn't seen the light of day since college and had a seamstress make two holes in it just big enough to fit the pumping shields through. It worked! And the added benefit? My husband found the effect incredibly sexy.

— PAM, ANCHORAGE, ALASKA

Chapter 3

ANSWERING YOUR
QUESTIONS

New moms love company—especially when it comes to breastfeeding. Get two moms together and it's just a matter of minutes before they start swapping war stories. Everyone has questions to ask and tales to tell about unsympathetic hospital nurses, leaking breasts, public breastfeeding, and, yes, sex with your enhanced anatomy.

Here's a true-or-false breastfeeding quiz to provide fuel for your tête-à-têtes. It will separate myth from reality and answer the questions that are keeping you up at night (as if the baby isn't already doing a good enough job of that!).

(1) Breasts can be too big or too small to feed a baby. True or false? *False.* You can breastfeed whether your cup size is AA or DDD. Breast size is determined by the amount of fat in your breasts and has nothing to do with the amount of milk-producing tissue.

(2) You might not make enough milk to feed your baby. True or false? *It depends.* At some point, every mom worries that she doesn't have enough milk to feed her baby. So here are a few things to keep in mind. As long as your baby gains weight and pees and poops, everything is probably fine. The key is that milk supply depends on stimulation. The more your baby sucks and swallows, the more milk you'll make. Babies who are sleepy, premature, or jaundiced sometimes don't suck enough. Additionally, your own pain and stress can impede milk production.

If a doctor or lactation consultant determines that your milk supply really is low, there are ways to increase production. For instance, you can encourage your baby to suck and swallow by holding him naked against your bare stomach and tickling his cheeks and feet. You can also use a breast pump between feedings to provide added stimulation for your breasts. There are even herbal and prescription remedies for increasing milk supply.

From the Mouths of Moms

Our son still wasn't back up to his birth weight at his two-week doctor's visit. So, over the next few weeks, my husband and I tried everything. He wouldn't stay awake at the breast, so we would rub and move him around. We even put a wet washcloth on every part of his body. But we had limited success. We could be at it for an hour and he'd only suckle for 10 to 15 minutes. In addition to breastfeeding, we were giving him supplements of breast milk or formula through a bottle, a syringe, and even a supplemental nutrition system. To make matters worse, he wasn't eating often enough to stimulate adequate milk production for me. I spent several weeks trying to make up the difference by pumping, taking fenugreek and blessed thistle, and talking to lactation consultants. I even resorted to acupuncture. Then, finally, it all came together. He was back to his birth weight by one month. He's eight weeks now, and he gained six ounces last week. I still worry that he's not getting enough, but I'm glad we stayed the course, and it all seems worth it!

— ANN, DES MOINES, IOWA

(3) If you've had surgery to reduce or enlarge your breasts, you won't be able to breastfeed. True or false? *False.* Women can breastfeed after surgery, but it can be a challenge if the surgery removed glandular tissue or damaged the milk ducts or nerves. Talk with your doctor or a lactation consultant, who will most likely tell you to give breastfeeding a try. Monitor the baby's weight and track the number of wet diapers to make sure she's getting enough to eat. If you have to, you can always use bottles of formula to supplement your nursing. Also, silicone implants are generally considered to be compatible with breastfeeding.

(4) Beer can help increase your milk supply. True or false? *True (at least anecdotally).* Some women swear by a glass of dark beer to increase their milk production. Research is inconclusive, but as long as you don't go overboard, one beer can't hurt (see number 5, below).

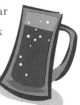

(5) You can't have caffeine or alcohol when you're breastfeeding. True or false? *True and false.* When you were pregnant, everything you ate ended up in your baby's system. Now you have a little more leeway—but moderation is the key! Caffeine can impact some babies, so keep it

to a minimum. Don't have a cup of coffee right before feeding a baby who should be sleeping. As for alcohol, the answers are sometimes conflicting. The general consensus is that you can have one to two drinks per week. Even the American Academy of Pediatrics says alcohol is fine in moderation. Your best bet is to breastfeed your baby before drinking; limit yourself to one drink; and wait a few hours for the alcohol to leave your body before feeding again. You don't have to pump and dump. On the other hand, the March of Dimes says breastfeeding moms should never drink alcohol because it can inhibit the flow of breast milk and even delay a baby's learning to walk and crawl. So, ultimately, it's up to you to decide what makes you most comfortable.

(6) **You need to avoid certain foods while breastfeeding. True or false?** *True and false.* When you were pregnant, your doctor may have told you to avoid deli meats and unpasteurized cheeses (because of bacteria) as well as certain fish (because of mercury). Now that you're breastfeeding, a few restrictions remain:

- Avoid unpasteurized cheeses and deli meats for the first week after giving birth.
- The U.S. Food and Drug Administration recommends staying away from fish that can contain mercury. Do not

From the Mouths of Moms

I accidentally discovered the milk-producing power of beer after a night at Sully's, our local joint. I had a burger and a Guinness, and the next day, my breasts were practically exploding. I didn't think anything of it until a week later when we went to Sully's again, and I ordered the same thing. Next day, same phenomenon with my milk supply. I drank a Guinness a day for the rest of the time I breastfed.

— MEREDITH, PROVIDENCE, RHODE ISLAND

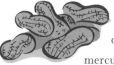 eat shark, swordfish, king mackerel, or tilefish. Albacore tuna contains more mercury than canned light tuna.

- Avoid peanuts if the baby, or any family member, has peanut or other food allergies, asthma or eczema.
- Dairy products can upset some breastfeeding infants, so eliminate dairy only if you think your baby has a problem.

(7) **You can continue to breastfeed if you are sick. True or false?** *It depends.* If you have a cold or the flu, not only *can* you breastfeed, you *should.* Your milk will contain antibodies that will help protect your baby from getting sick. Certain

conditions, of course, are much more serious. Moms in developed countries who have HIV should not breastfeed since the disease can be passed through milk. Also, if a mom has herpes or syphilis sores on one breast, she should feed from the other side. As always, consult your doctor.

(8)　You can't take any medicine while you're breastfeeding. True or false? *False.* Many medicines, such as Advil, Tylenol, some antibiotics, and some decongestants, are fine. But other medications can harm a baby or decrease your milk supply. It's best to run everything by your doctor. Note, too, that your doctor's advice may change as your baby gets older. To do your own research, check out Thomas Hale's book and the Web site Toxnet (see "Resources," page 153).

(9)　You can't get pregnant if you're breastfeeding. True or false? *It depends.* Breastfeeding can stop your body from menstruating for a while, but it's not always birth control. Unless you're comfortable with the idea of having kids very close together in age, you'll want to use some form of contraceptives. If you do want to rely on breastfeeeding as birth control (the Lactational Amenorrhea Method), you must answer "no" to all of the following:

· Have you resumed menstruating?

· Is your baby more than six months old?

- Are you supplementing regularly or going long
  stretches without breastfeeding (3 hours during
  the day and 6 hours at night)?

(10) You can't take oral contraceptives while breastfeeding.
True or false? *False.* Pills that contain estrogen have
been shown to decrease milk supply, but a progesterone-
only pill is fine. Your doctor will probably talk to you
about birth control at your first postpartum checkup.

(11) If you stop breastfeeding, it's possible to start again.
True or false? *True.* With a big dose of patience, it may
be possible to start breastfeeding again. Moms may want
to do so if there is a shortage of food due to an emergency
or after being separated from the baby for an extended
period. Relactation is easier if your baby is younger than
four months and you initially had a good milk supply, but
it's not impossible with older babies. Pumping, frequent
feedings, and taking certain supplements can get the ball
rolling again. Some moms may also use a device called
a supplemental nursing system (SNS); the mom wears
a container of milk around her neck, and a tube leads
to her nipple. The baby sucks on her breast and the tube
at the same time, thereby ensuring a supply of milk
and nipple stimulation simultaneously.

From the Mouths of Moms

One of my more embarrassing moments was when my older daughter was three weeks old. I felt like I'd been stuck in the house for an eternity. My husband came home from work one evening and invited me out for ice cream. My mother stayed at home with the baby, and I was absolutely thrilled to go out on a mini-date. We drove to the nearest ice cream shop and stood in a long line. Much to my chagrin, I looked down and realized that I had forgotten a breast pad—I was leaking breast milk all over my T-shirt! I told my husband I'd wait for my ice cream in the car, and that was the end of my big outing.

— ELLEN, BETHESDA, MARYLAND

(12) **You can breastfeed a baby you adopt. True or false?** *True.* That may come as a surprise, but with the help of a doctor and a lactation consultant, you may be able to lactate even if you haven't given birth. It's pretty hard to produce all the milk that a baby needs, and some women will obviously have more success than others. You'll probably need to use a breast pump and take certain medications or herbal supplements to stimulate milk production. A supplemental nursing system can help as well (see number 11, above).

(13) You can get human milk from a breast-milk bank if you're unable to breastfeed your baby. True or false?

True. Since the early twentieth century, milk banks have helped babies whose moms were unable to breastfeed. The first milk bank in the United States opened in Boston in 1919. Today there are eleven milk banks in the United States and Canada that store human breast milk from carefully screened donors. To get milk, you'll need a doctor's prescription or hospital purchase order. If you want to donate milk, contact the Human Milk Banking Association of North America (see "Resources," page 153).

Mama Data

Thousands of years ago, wet-nursing was quite common. In ancient Greece, Rome, and Egypt, wealthy families hired wet nurses to breast-feed their children. Wet nurses also cared for children abandoned at birth. This pattern continued in Europe through the Middle Ages and Renaissance. Wealthy families often sent their infants to live with wet nurses, and hospitals for abandoned babies employed wet nurses. Poor women typically nursed their own children. By the late seventeenth century, however, medical professionals began to encourage mothers to breastfeed their own babies.

(14) If you both breastfeed and bottle-feed, your baby may experience "nipple confusion" or "flow preference." True or false? *Depends on the baby.* Some professionals believe that giving a bottle or pacifier to a breastfed baby can cause "nipple confusion" and thus interfere with breastfeeding. Here's one way to look at it—just as you're probably pretty set in your ways, your baby can quickly become a creature of habit. Breastfeeding and bottle-feeding require different tongue and sucking motions. The amount of flow from a bottle is also different from that from a breast, so it can be hard for the baby to learn a new technique. But every baby is different. Some will switch back and forth easily between the two. Others might refuse the bottle if they're accustomed to the boob, or vice versa. If you're trying to do both, wait at least three or four weeks after your baby is born before you introduce a bottle. Then cross your fingers and hope that your kiddo will go with the flow.

(15) Breastfeeding ruins the shape of your breasts. True or false? *False.* Your breasts will never quite look the same. It's sad, but true. But breastfeeding isn't the culprit. Pregnancy, heredity, and weight are to blame for changing the shape of your breasts.

Mama Data

If you think your bottles, breast pump, and nipple shields are marvels of the twentieth century, think again. Similar devices have been around for centuries. The earliest "bottles" were horns, vases, and jugs. Writers in the sixteenth century describe "breast pumps"—a glass cup that a woman placed on her breast and an attached tube she sucked on to relieve engorgement and express milk. In the same period, women sometimes used "nipple shields" made of wood or metal.

(16) You need to wean your baby if you get pregnant. True or false? *Maybe.* There is no clear-cut answer here; it's really up to you and your doctor. Some doctors say that it's fine to continue nursing while you're pregnant. Others will counsel you to stop to ensure the growing baby is adequately nourished or if you are at risk of preterm labor.

(17) You won't be able to breastfeed if you have inverted nipples. True or false? *False.* Some women's nipples don't stick out much and may appear "flat" or even inverted. If this sounds familiar, don't worry. With a little patience, you can help your baby latch on. Most likely, your baby's sucking motion

will draw out your nipple. If not, try pumping or using
a nipple shield, a silicone nipple that sits directly on your
breasts. As your baby sucks, the milk comes out through
holes in the shield. Eventually you'll remove the shield, and
your baby will do well without it. If you're having a hard
time, talk to a lactation consultant (see page 56).

(18)   You can develop an infection in your breast while
breastfeeding. True or False? *True.* Of course, not
everyone ends up with an infection, but it can happen.
Mastitis, an inflammation of the breast tissue, can make
you feel like you have the flu. You can have a fever and
chills, and your breasts can feel hot, tender, and swollen.
If your doctor determines that you have an infection,
she might prescribe an antibiotic. Some commonsense
remedies can help, too. Sleep, eat, and drink lots of water.
Apply warm compresses to your breasts to increase
circulation, followed by cold compresses to reduce swelling.
Reduce pressure on your chest by sleeping without a bra
and lying on your back or on the side of your body that
isn't sore. Feed the baby frequently on the infected side
to keep the milk flowing and to avoid a plugged duct.
Worst-case senario: an infection can develop into an
abscess, a localized infection that a doctor may need
to open surgically and drain (see page 58).

(19) Your baby can decide to go on a breastfeeding strike. **True or false?** *True.* For a variety of reasons, a baby who has been feeding well can suddenly refuse to nurse. He could be teething or have a stuffed nose, ear infection, or yeast infection. Or maybe he's reacting to a change in routine, stress in the household, or being left with a babysitter. Not to fear—you can fix the situation. Have your pediatrician make sure the baby is healthy, then focus on spending a lot of time with him. Try feeding the baby when he's sleepy, or even when he's already asleep.

(20) A lump in your breast while breastfeeding is cause for concern. **True or false?** *It depends.* Women often develop breast lumps when breastfeeding. A lump can be caused by a plugged duct, an infection, or a benign tumor or cyst. The lump will often go away once you've fed your baby. Hot compresses can help, too. If it's still there in a week, see your doctor. It's rare for these lumps to be cancerous. In fact, studies have found that breastfeeding can reduce a woman's risk of getting cancer. But take any lump seriously. You can develop breast cancer while breastfeeding (see page 57).

From the Mouths of Moms

My last bout of mastitis occurred when I flew with my newborn from Germany to the United States to hunt for a new house. Surprise, surprise. With the time change, house hunt, and stress, I allowed the feeding cycles to lapse and I got run-down. Bam! I got hit with mastitis. I was alone in a hotel room with my baby when I was at my worst. I was so sick with a fever that I couldn't even fathom leaving the room to pick up my antibiotic prescription. I thought taking a bath might help bring down my fever. While waiting for the tub to fill, the baby fell asleep, and then I did as well. Before I knew it, the bathroom and part of the hotel room were flooded. Imagine my embarrassment when I had to call the maintenance folks to save me from myself. The guy assured me that he'd seen worse. I don't know if he meant worse floods or worse visions of a mother in stress.

— MEG, LARCHMONT, NEW YORK

Breastfeeding hurts. True or false? *True and false.* If the baby is latched on well and sucking properly, breastfeeding shouldn't be painful. But it's not always the most comfortable activity in the world. During the first few weeks, as the two of you are learning your pas de deux, your breasts might be a little tender. But if you have pain with a capital P, then something more serious is probably going on. The worst-case scenarios are cracked and bleeding nipples, engorged breasts, plugged ducts, and mastitis. Fortunately, you can fix these problems, and the pain will go away. Just get help from your doctor and/or a lactation consultant. And get help fast. The longer you wait, the worse the pain will be.

(22) **You can sometimes feel sexually aroused while breastfeeding. True or false?** *True.* OK, so that may sound a little weird, but, really, it's perfectly normal to sometimes get aroused while nursing. Here's the reason: The body releases the hormones oxytocin and prolactin during both breastfeeding and sex. So if you're feeling a little turned on, not to fear. There's nothing wrong with you. Just enjoy. If it's really bothering you, take a break from the feeding and try again a little later.

(23) **You have to sterilize breast-pump equipment and bottles. True or false?** *False.* You'll hear lots of different opinions on this one. Basically, warm, soapy water is fine, and every once in a while you may want to put the parts in boiling water (see page 59).

(24) **Pacifiers aren't good for breastfed babies. True or false?**
It depends. Pacifiers are a hot-button issue. People in the
antipacifier camp say pacifiers can mask hunger cues.
Those in the propacifier camp say pacifiers are good
if your baby needs to suck long after she's done eating.
The American Academy of Pediatrics (AAP) recommends
pacifiers during sleep for the first year to reduce the risk
of Sudden Infant Death Syndrome (SIDS). For breastfed
babies, the AAP advises waiting until the baby
is one month old and breastfeeding is well
established before using a pacifier. If the
baby refuses the pacifier, don't force it.

(25) **Wet-nursing and cross nursing are another way for your
baby to get breast milk. True or false?** *True, but it's not
always safe.* Hundreds of years ago, moms commonly hired
wet nurses to feed their babies, but that practice has all but
disappeared in the United States. As for cross nursing, or
casually breastfeeding another woman's baby, there's no
way to know how many people are doing this. La Leche
League advises against both practices because the person
feeding your baby could have a communicable disease.
Additionally, milk from another mother may not have the
precise composition that your baby needs at any given age.

From the Mouths of Moms

When my sister's son was one month old, she laughingly put off my request to nurse him. But one day she had to go out, and she asked me to watch the baby. Of course, I nursed him when he started fussing. When she returned, she said, "You put him on the minute my car was out of the driveway, didn't you?" She didn't really mind, but she did chalk it up to me being a weirdo. Then, the next day, she came bursting through the door and shoved the baby into my arms. "Here!" she said, "He's been driving me crazy, nursing all night long! He's all yours!"

— HELENA, MAPLEWOOD, NEW JERSEY

Chapter 4

TRICKS OF THE TRADE

There was probably a time when you considered getting a perm, learning to drive, or living with your boyfriend to be a major lifestyle change. Yes, those were some big milestones. But *nothing* compares to having a baby. As soon as your bundle of joy arrives, you realize that your life will now forever be broken into two distinct categories—Before Baby (B.B.) and After Baby (A.B.). Suddenly *you* are responsible for the care and feeding of an utterly dependent human being. A human being who is very hungry—and whose food is produced inside your own body!

There's little doubt you'll settle into your own A.B. routine, but to nudge you along, here are some tricks of the trade for sleep, fashion, work, and all your other newfound responsibilities.

Sleep

Most newborns feed every two or three hours. Unfortunately, the two-hour countdown starts when you *begin* the feeding rather than when you end it. In other words, if you fed the baby at 9:00, you do it again at 11:00. For at least the first few weeks, this goes on twenty-four hours a day!

How long can you keep up this crazy schedule before you collapse from exhaustion? The good news is that it won't last forever. In the beginning, it's basically about survival. After a few weeks, babies go for longer stretches—three to four hours—between feedings. Then, after a few months, most babies can sleep through the night without waking to eat. (Of course, every baby has different needs, so get your pediatrician's input.) Here are some tips for surviving those first few months.

❀ *Divide and conquer.* Divvy up responsibilities with your spouse. You do feedings. He does diapers.

❀ *Go to bed early.* No more *Letterman* for you.

❀ *Nap when the baby naps.* Every little bit helps.

❀ *Keep a journal.* A brief log of naps, diaper changes, feeding times, and sides that you fed on will help you keep things straight despite your postpartum fog. (Journaling is also useful if your baby ever needs to take medicine at certain times of day.) Stop if the note-taking seems stressful, tedious, or unnecessary.

❀ ***Accept all offers of help.*** Let friends bring over dinner.

❀ ***Let the housework go.*** Forget the laundry and dishes. Get used to those dust bunnies under your bed.

❀ ***Hire help if you can afford it.*** When the mess gets really bad, bring in a housekeeper. Consider hiring a childcare expert to help take care of the baby.

❀ ***Pump.*** Once you've spent a month or so establishing a good milk supply and breastfeeding schedule, pump milk so that your husband can take care of one of the feedings. Don't forget—if your baby is taking a bottle but you aren't pumping, your supply may drop.

❀ ***Co-sleep. Bring the baby into your bed.*** She'll wake up to eat and fall right back to sleep. But be careful. There's a serious risk that a baby could suffocate or get hurt. Avoid co-sleeping if one parent has been drinking or is heavily medicated, overweight, or excessively tired.

❀ ***Use a bassinet in your room.*** If the baby is next to your bed, you'll hear her right away and won't have to go too far to feed her.

From the Mouths of Moms

After a week of conscientious breastfeeding, I realized I might be doomed. I was exhausted, my son was starving, and the pediatrician said the baby had lost weight. I had a lactation consultant visit my house for additional "training." Ultimately, I decided to supplement with a couple of bottles. My baby was satisfied. And though I had hoped to experience the Zen-like state so many nursing women refer to, the only state of nirvana I achieved was finally giving in to hiring a night nurse. I only had to get into bed, turn off the baby monitor, and kiss my husband goodnight. *It was glorious!*

— MOIRA, DENVER, COLORADO

✿ *Train an older baby to sleep through the night.*

Many babies can sleep through the night by the time they are about three months old. If yours is still waking to eat, you can continue feedings, or if you prefer, start to nudge her to sleep longer stretches. Ask your pediatrician for advice. There are many different philosophies about "sleep training." (That's a whole book in itself!)

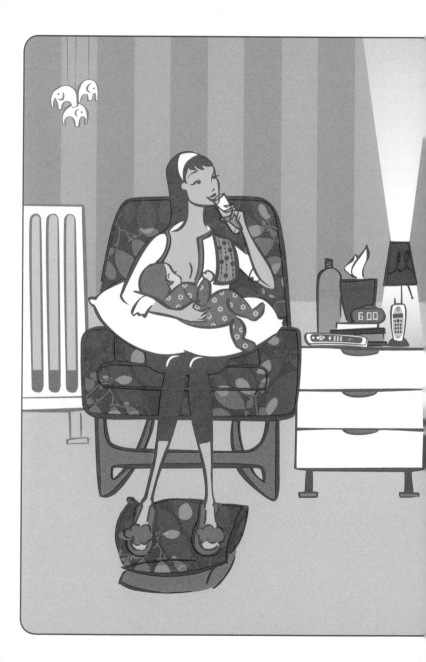

Essential Props

Breastfeeding in the comfort and quiet of your own home can be quite relaxing and, dare I say, serene. Someday your baby will even smile at you between gulps, and you'll absolutely melt.

To make these moments a little more sublime, you'll want some key items within reach. Seriously, keep these things nearby. You will not want to get up to retrieve the remote control once your baby is contentedly eating away.

(1) **Footstool.** Buy a "nursing stool," a footrest specifically designed to prop your legs at a comfortable angle and support your lower back. But any old footrest will do. Try a phone book or even a box of toys. Then sit back and relax.

(2) **Rocking chair.** You might find the rocking motion soothing to both you and the baby.

(3) **Pillows.** Put a pillow on your lap to raise the baby closer to your chest. Pillows under your elbows can also relieve tension in your back and arms.

(4) **Burp cloth**. This one's pretty self-explanatory.

(5) **CD player or iPod:** You'll need all the help you can get to stay awake. Plus, you can let a recording sing the lullabies for you.

(6) **Television remote control**. What could be better than giving yourself the license to watch TV in the middle of the day? Figure out the closed-captioning function if you don't want to distract your baby. This is also the perfect excuse to get a digital video recorder so that you can watch whatever you want, whenever you want. It's likely you'll have trouble watching an entire show during one feeding. Sometimes it can take days to get through one hour of programming.

(7) **Water.** It is important to stay well hydrated. Dark yellow urine and constipation are signs of dehydration.

(8) **Food.** Avoid hot foods or dishes that require utensils. Instead, have something neat and compact. Crumbs have a way of getting stuck in the fat rolls under your baby's chin.

(9) **Cordless telephone.** This item is virtually a necessity. If it's not right next to you, it will definitely ring the minute the baby latches on. A headset is also helpful to avoid a stiff neck. But beware: Before you know it, your baby will try to grab the phone and start dialing!

(10) **Something to read.** Forget *War and Peace*—all books should weigh less than your baby. Magazines are easy to hold, but newspaper pages can be hard to turn.

(11) **Tissues.** Make sure you always have a tissue tucked into your shirtsleeve, grandma-style.

Multitasking

It's normal to feel overwhelmed, not only by the baby, but also by your unanswered e-mails, unwritten thank-you notes, unpaid bills, and even your unkempt hair and fingernails. But consider putting your compulsive side to rest for a little while. Try to look at breastfeeding as your ticket to sitting down and taking a breather. For at least twenty minutes a pop, you can ignore the outside world. You've got something much more important to do.

Fashion

Celebrity moms have done the rest of us a disservice. We see magazine pictures of Gwyneth Paltrow looking pregnant, radiant, and wearing the latest in maternity wear. Then just one month later we're poring over photos of her toting the darling "Apple" of her eye, back to looking as chic and svelte as ever. And you? You're sporting the same sweatpants you wore yesterday, you haven't washed your hair in three days, and you've got spit-up stains on your shoulder. You think to yourself, where did I go wrong?

Let's be realistic. Comparing yourself to celebrities is absurd. So stop *right now*. Ignore the magazines and TV shows. These women have personal trainers to whip them back into shape, chefs to cook them healthy meals, and full-time nannies to take care of their "celebu-tots" while they go to the spa. They also have the money—and stylists—to buy the perfect wardrobe for both pre- and post-baby. Most important, they hide from the paparazzi until they're ready for prime time.

So what's a mere mortal to do? Accept that getting back in shape takes a while. You won't fit into your old pre-pregnancy clothes right away. It took 40 weeks for you to put on those 35+ pounds, and it will take you a while to get rid of them, too.

But here's some *really* good news—breastfeeding can help you lose weight because it burns roughly 500 calories per day. It might take several months, but there *will* come a day when you can once again wear your favorite jeans.

So what does all this mean for your wardrobe? How can you look as cute as your tyke, who seems to have a new outfit every day? Try these tips on for size:

✿ *Work backward through your clothes.* What you wore on your way up the scale, wear on the way back down.

✿ *Buy staple items that you can wear repeatedly without people noticing.* For instance, you can wear the same jeans or black pants day in and day out if you change your top. A few T-shirts, turtlenecks, and sweaters are good basics.

✿ *Accessorize.* Go for the latest "it" handbag or piece of jewelry. At least then you won't look like you've been hibernating for the past ten months.

✿ *Buy new shoes.* No guilt here, my friend. You'll probably need the new footwear since your feet may have grown when you were pregnant.

❀ ***Buy some sexy nursing bras.*** Lace. Leopard print. Bright
red silk! Believe it or not, you can find some pretty sexy nursing
bras. So go for a bit of glitz. It will be a welcome change from
your everyday nursing bras that are most likely grey from
constant washings.

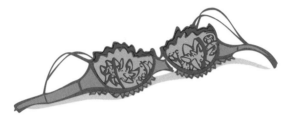

❀ ***Find a few pieces that allow you to discreetly breastfeed
in public.*** Basically, you want to wear something that you
can pull up without exposing too much skin. A poncho,
shawl, or scarf is a safe bet over any outfit. There are even
wraps and tops specifically designed for the nursing mom.
If you aren't going to splurge for new clothes, here's a good
combo: Wear a button-down blouse over a tank top.

From the Mouths of Moms

When my son was born, a lactation consultant at the hospital told me she couldn't meet with us until later because she had to go eat dinner. My son, born at 5 pounds 11 ounces, had dropped to 4 pounds 14 ounces and wasn't nursing because he was premature and didn't latch well. I looked at my husband and said, "Did she just say what I thought she did?" I'm a nurse, and I was furious at her. We ended up finding a private lactation consultant who helped us so much.

— JENNIFER, ATLANTA, GEORGIA

Who Can Help?

One of the biggest challenges of being a mom, and a breastfeeding mom at that, is getting help with breastfeeding questions. Who's the best person to call for practical tips? Moral support? Medical problems? Consult the list below to determine whose number to dial.

✿ *Lactation Consultant.* She is the goddess of all things booby. Make sure that yours has the title "IBCLC," for International Board Certified Lactation Consultant.

❀ ***Pediatrician.*** Although she can monitor the success of your breastfeeding by charting your child's growth, she may not be hands-on like a lactation consultant. Chances are, however, she knows a thing or two about breastfeeding. After all, she does see little babies every day, all day.

❀ ***Obstetrician.*** This doctor brought your baby safely into the world. Can she help you with breastfeeding? Maybe, maybe not. It's definitely worth asking. At a minimum, she can refer you to a lactation consultant.

❀ ***Midwife.*** She may have provided your medical care during pregnancy and birth. She's not an M.D., but she's gone through a rigorous education and certification process. Does she know anything about breastfeeding? Ask her a few questions, and then decide for yourself.

❀ ***Hospital Nurse.*** When she pops into your recovery room, hopefully she can answer some of your questions. If you feel you want a specialist, ask to see a lactation consultant who works at the hospital. And one more thing: If you don't want hospital nurses or doctors giving your baby formula or a pacifier, put a sign on the baby's bassinet that says "Mom's milk only. No bottles or pacifiers, please. Get my mom if I wake up."

From the Mouths of Moms

When my daughter Adele was born, I was quite surprised by the challenges of nursing. I was prepared for exhaustion, but not for the soreness and latching issues. Fortunately, I had a postpartum doula who showed me nursing techniques and encouraged me to keep going when I felt overwhelmed. My husband was also very supportive. We still laugh about the early days when he would hold Adele and try to position her on my breast. We were in nursing boot camp together. I continued to nurse Adele until she was nine months old. She was sick only once during that time, and now she's a strong, healthy, and happy girl. What more could a Mom want? Well . . . I did lose a dress size.

— ANDREA, CHICAGO, ILLINOIS

✿ *Postpartum Doula.* She will provide both emotional and practical support (childcare, cooking, and light housekeeping) once you're home with the baby. She may know a good deal about breastfeeding since she's probably seen just about everything.

✿ **"Baby Nurse."** Some moms hire a "baby nurse" to care for their newborns at home. These baby nurses may even stay around the clock to help at night. While many have years of experience caring for newborns, make sure you check credentials. Not all are registered nurses. And if they are giving you advice about breastfeeding, make sure it resonates with you. Don't feel forced into following a prescribed feeding schedule. Feed your baby when she's hungry, even if she just ate ten minutes ago.

✿ **Spouse or Partner.** Too bad Mother Nature insisted on a division of labor. If men could lactate, then at least you'd get a little more sleep. Even so, your spouse can probably lend a hand. After all, he's pretty familiar with this part of your anatomy, and with an outsider's perspective he may be able to help you position the baby on your breast. At the very least, he can get you a glass of water and an extra pillow. Once you're done feeding, he can burp and diaper the baby.

✿ **Your Friend.** Has she had a baby of her own yet? If not, don't be surprised if she doesn't really believe that for the past month you haven't slept for more than three hours at a stretch. Would you have believed it before you had a baby? If she has had a baby, she'll know why you haven't called her since you got home from the hospital. If she gives you breastfeeding advice, be aware that what worked for her may not work for you.

❖ ***Moms, Grandmas, Aunts, Sisters, and Cousins.*** The women in your family will have different levels of expertise. It's quite possible that your mom and grandmother never breastfed since it was less common in past generations.

❖ ***Breastfeeding Support Group.*** You may have never met these women before, but listening to their stories might make you realize you aren't all alone. Somewhere out there, there's another mother up at 3 A.M. feeding her baby, too. Your local hospital may run a support group.

❖ ***Online Communities.*** Many Web sites and blogs are devoted to breastfeeding. You can post questions that will be answered by both experts and other moms. For a list of suggested sites, check the "Resources" section (page 153).

Going Back to Work?

As moms, we all work. Whether you're a working mom (WM), a stay-at-home mom (SAHM), or a work-at-home mom (WAHM), you have a full-time job. But one thing is certain—when you work outside the home, your breastfeeding assignment is a bit more complicated. It's unlikely you can regularly bring your baby to work, so you'll be pumping like it's going out of style. Here's some advice on becoming a breastfeeding WM.

✿ *Train your baby to take both bottle and boob.* Babies can be notoriously picky about how they get their meals. To make sure your babe will accept two types of nipples, start giving her a bottle when she's three or four weeks old.

✿ *Breastfeed before you leave for work and as soon as you get home.* You'll get one last snuggle before you head out the door and another as soon as you walk in.

✿ *Tell your boss you need to pump while you're at work.* Only you know best how to handle this discussion.

From the Mouths of Moms

I used to pump at work during very long conference calls. This required wedging the bottles against the desk so I could take notes while the pump was going. I would mute the phone so the others couldn't hear that whirring sound. Inevitably, I would be midpump when I was called upon to speak. I'd have to turn off the pump as quickly as possible, move the bottles so they wouldn't spill, press the "unmute" button, and try to sound professional and cool. Talk about juggling!

— LEAH, SEATTLE, WASHINGTON

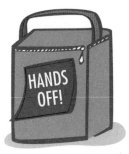

❀ *Arrange for a private pumping location.* If you're fortunate enough to have your own office, simply close the door. If it doesn't lock, find a way to make sure that people knock before entering. Post a "Do Not Disturb" sign or have a colleague run interference. If you work in a cubicle or an open space, ask your boss to designate a lactation room.

❀ *Time your pumping sessions to coincide with times when the baby eats at home.* Doing so will ensure that you produce enough milk.

❀ *Leave your pump at work.* Just carry a cooler with the pumped milk back and forth each day.

❀ *Store the milk in a cooler bag in the office refrigerator.* Post a "Hands Off" sign. If there isn't a refrigerator, pack the cooler with ice packs. It should be fine for the day.

Chapter 5

BREASTFEEDING
ETIQUETTE

***Breastfeeding is emerging from homes across
the country to find a new place in the public eye.***
While previous generations of women rarely breastfed in
public, many of today's moms are bold and self-confident.
They refuse to spend all day cooped up at home just
because the baby needs to eat every few hours. With
discretion, they hit the road toting their portable
kitchen—their breasts.

Of course, not everyone is comfortable feeding in
public. Some moms will do it only in cases of emergency,
and even then only in places where no one can see.
Not everyone is a "lactivist," a breastfeeding activist,
ready to stage a public "nurse-in" at a Starbucks or
Victoria's Secret. Some women prefer the comfort and
quiet of their couch at home, and, even there, they may
retreat to another room if nosy relatives are visiting.

If you do accidentally flash a little boob while you're
out and about, don't worry. It's not illegal to breastfeed
in public. In fact, depending on what state you're in, the
law may protect your right to do so. There are states that
exempt breastfeeding mothers from indecency laws, states
that protect breastfeeding in public and private areas,
states that require employers to make accommodations
for women who need to pump, and even states that excuse

breastfeeding women from jury duty. If you want to know how your state handles the issue, check out the National Conference of State Legislatures (see "Resources," page 153). In addition, a federal law says that you can breastfeed on all federal property. Courthouse or post office, anyone?

Even if the law is on your side, you may not always get a warm reception from the public at large. Public breastfeeding can still stir up quite a bit of controversy. We may not think twice about a half-naked woman on an advertising billboard or a bikini-clad supermodel in a sports magazine, but when it comes to an infant hiding under her mom's shirt to eat lunch, some people get all worked up. Breastfeeding women are kicked off airplanes and asked to leave stores and restaurants. They're subjected to unsolicited comments and stares. It's no wonder some moms don't want to breastfeed anywhere but home.

From the Mouths of Moms

I breastfed everywhere—restaurants, airports, airplanes, the zoo, a street curb in Shanghai, the Paris metro, walking down the street. My best story? I breastfed while on an exercise machine! Bennett was quietly sleeping in his car seat, so I took him with me to the hotel exercise room to sleep while I worked out. He slept quietly beside me for the first 10 minutes, then woke up and clearly needed to eat. I was the only person in the small workout room, so I decided to go for it. I was on the type of bike that allows you to recline and peddle hands-free, so while I biked, he ate. It worked great. But boy did we surprise the man who got on the bike next to us.

— ELIZABETH, SAN FRANCISCO, CALIFORNIA

As you contemplate whether to breastfeed on a park bench or listen to your child scream until you get home, know that you aren't alone in your dilemma. Every day millions of women are making the same choice. And even if you do get some strange looks and comments, you'll also probably get some friendly smiles and encouraging remarks. Heck, you may even make friends with another mom and find a future playmate for your baby.

To Feed or Not to Feed?

Since there isn't an Emily Post guide to public breastfeeding, you'll have to make up your own rules. In most cases, that means using commonsense. If it seems like you're pushing the envelope just a little too much, think twice. For instance, afternoon tea at the Four Seasons with your great-aunt probably isn't the best time to feed your baby. Maybe it would be better to excuse yourself and go to the lobby.

In general, a little creativity will go a long way. Shopping for clothes? Sit on the floor between racks of clothing. Taking a road trip? Try the backseat of your car. Here's a list of mom-tested breastfeeding places as well as suggestions on how to handle the need to feed.

Airplane: Being on a plane with a baby is not a lot of fun. You're stressed out, the baby is cranky, and nearby passengers are begging the flight attendant for new seat assignments. You might be leery of feeding while stuck so close to other travelers, but if it stops your baby from crying, those around you will likely be quite thankful. Breastfeeding will also help relieve some of the pressure your baby may feel in his ears due to the altitude. Go for it!

Bathtub: Caution—slippery when wet! It might seem efficient to breastfeed and wash leaky diapers and cheesy burps off both you and your baby at the same time, but it's not as great as it sounds. Wet babies are slippery. Very slippery. If you insist on trying this, get your spouse to spot you.

Beach or pool: If a bikini is okay, why not a breastfeeding baby? For propriety's sake, and sun protection, put a towel over the baby and your shoulder. And, of course, don't forget sunblock and a hat for the baby. A huge umbrella is another way to block the sun. If the baby is less than six months old, check with your pediatrician about whether she can wear sunscreen.

Bookstore: A quiet, book-filled environment can be soothing for both you and your baby. Camp out in a neglected aisle where few people tread, and settle in among the shelves.

Bus: Buses follow the same principle as airplanes (see page III). No one wants to spend an entire ride listening to a miserable child. Feed your baby, and he'll quiet down. He might even go to sleep, giving you a chance to catch your breath.

Car: At some point, whether on a long road trip or a short jaunt to the grocery store, your baby will scream inconsolably from the backseat. If you determine that it's food he wants, you have a choice: Either pull over and breastfeed, or continue driving and listen to your baby work himself into a sweaty lather.

Parking lots are your safest bet. Look for a spot on the edge of the lot, where there isn't much traffic. A parking spot on the side of the street is less safe since you have to take the baby out of his car seat while other cars are whizzing by. Avoid pulling off to the side of a highway; wait for the next exit and find a parking lot.

If you're a passenger in the backseat with the baby, you might be tempted to try to lean over his car seat to stick a boob in his mouth. But unless you're a contortionist, it probably won't work. Keep your seatbelt on, the baby in the car seat, and ask the driver to make a pit stop. Finally, don't even think about breastfeeding while driving.

Cinema: The movies are an excellent place to breastfeed. You can catch the latest flick (before it ends up on DVD) and your infant may happily oblige. Some movie theaters even run special movie times for moms and their babies. There is one major downside—changing diapers. Your choices are limited: (a) go to the bathroom and miss part of the movie; (b) change the baby on a popcorn- and candy-coated floor; (c) change the baby on a slanted, dark aisle; or (d) balance the baby on your lap or another folding seat. Also, as your baby gets older and more alert, he may want to watch the movie rather than eat and sleep.

Doctor's or Dentist's Office: A medical establishment seems like a suitable place to feed a baby. Ask the staff if you can use an empty examining room. If your baby starts crying during your exam, try feeding him. Your doctor has seen it all already. If you're in the waiting room, simply practice discretion.

From the Mouths of Moms

I couldn't believe it when my mother scolded me (gently, but conde-scendingly) for nursing my one-week-old at his baby shower. He was born three weeks early, so he arrived in time for his own party. My mother said, "I can see what you are doing and I myself don't mind, but the busboy might not like it." I was astounded. The busboy?

— KATY, BARRINGTON, RHODE ISLAND

Family Gatherings: Holidays, birthdays, graduations, and religious events pop up all year long, and you're not about to miss the party just because you're breastfeeding. Besides, everyone wants to see the baby. So what's a mom to do? On the one hand, you could say that the politeness principle applies. If the host will be offended or annoyed that you're breastfeeding in front of everyone, then perhaps you should find a private place. On the other hand, this is your family, and shouldn't you be able to be yourself? Maybe this is your chance to gently suggest that public breastfeeding is perfectly natural. Besides, you're nourishing the next generation on the family tree!

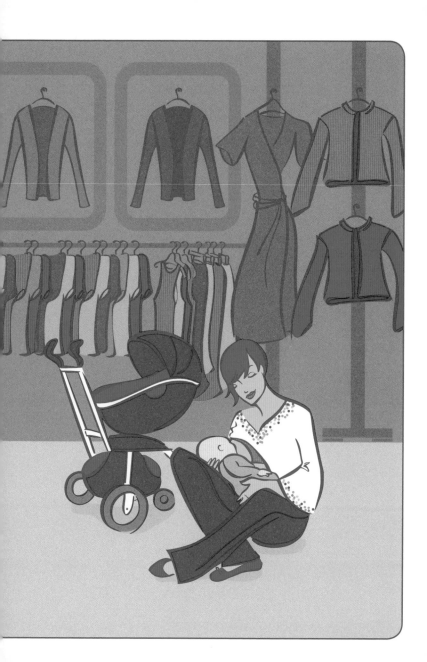

Federal Property (courthouses, museums, parks, post offices, and government buildings): Federal law protects a mom's right to breastfeed on any federal property where she is otherwise authorized to be. So, though it might not be the most comfortable place in the world, you can breastfeed at the post office.

Gym or Athletic Club: Find yourself walking past an athletic club when your baby is crying for a snack? Beg the people at the main desk to take pity on you and let you in (even if you don't have a membership). The sight of a little breast shouldn't be shocking to someone changing her clothes in the locker room.

Kitchen: Cooking while holding a baby? Bad, bad, bad idea. There's no upside to holding your baby while stirring a simmering sauce or dropping pasta into boiling water. The baby can wait a few minutes while you finish in the kitchen.

Library: Seek out a neglected aisle, give your baby lunch, and you'll ensure he doesn't break the no-talking rule.

Malls and Clothing Stores: Fitting rooms can give you a great deal of privacy and maybe even a real seat. Even if you're not trying something on, the look of desperation in your eyes will certainly melt the resolve of all but the most hardened salesperson. Just tell her you won't be in there too long, taking up precious changing space. She doesn't need to know that your kid can chow for a solid half hour!

From the Mouths of Moms

Before our son was born, my husband was pretty uncomfortable when friends breastfed in front of him. But I was amazed at how he transformed once we had Daniel. "Women should be able to breastfeed anywhere," he says now. He no longer views breasts (mine included) as sexual objects, but rather as imperative to the health and welfare of infants. I'm sure this is a common trait in men, but it still amazes me.

— SARAH, ALBANY, NEW YORK

Museum: Visiting a museum can ward off cabin fever after days and days of rain. But be forewarned. Seats are few and far between, and, when you find one, it will probably be smack in the middle of the room, without a back to lean against. Try the museum restaurant or coffee shop.

Office: It's unlikely that you'll take your baby to the office more than a couple of times. Sure, it's nice to show her off to your coworkers, but kids aren't exactly a welcome addition to most workplaces. Besides, do you really want everyone manhandling her? If you do take her in, the office environment will determine whether or not you'll want to breastfeed. If you're lucky, you can close and lock the door to a private office or conference room.

Park or Playground: The playground is bound to be a familiar stomping ground if you have an older child or you're hanging out with a friend who has older kids. If you have a toddler already, be prepared to chase after him while clutching the feeding infant to your chest. You may expose a little skin during this balancing act, but try not to feel too self-conscious. The playground is full of parents, grandparents, babysitters, and nannies who might feel sorry for you and offer to lend a helping hand.

Parties: Once upon a time, you headed out the door at 10 P.M. on a Saturday night. Now you're headed straight to bed. At some point, however, you're bound to go stir-crazy and consider toting your tot along with you to a party. If you do, and you stay for any length of time, you'll probably need to breastfeed. Just consider the crowd and the expectations of your host. At a low-key gathering of old friends, it might not be a big deal to socialize while feeding. If the scene is more uptight—such as a get-together of your parents' friends—then you'll probably want to retreat to another room. It might annoy you to feel like you're hiding, but just finish what you need to do and you'll be back with the gang soon enough.

Religious Service: Attending religious services may be an integral part of your life. But can you breastfeed while you're there? Only you can best answer that question, based on the standards of your community. If you do plan to feed while praying or listening to a sermon, consider wearing a scarf, shawl, or blanket over your shoulder and baby.

Restaurants and Coffee Shops: Breastfeeding burns calories, so it's likely that both you and your baby will be ravenous. Look for a table in the corner of the room where you'll feel comfortable. A table napkin can double as a burp cloth or cover-up.

Sports Stadium: If you're a mom so devoted to your favorite team that you're ready to indoctrinate your baby from day one, remember that you are just one of thousands in the stands. Everyone is watching the game, and they really don't care what you and your baby are doing. The people near you may be curious, but once they take a quick look, they'll probably go right back to keeping an eye on the action. You can always drape a team T-shirt over your shoulder.

Theaters and Concert Halls: These might be among your favorite places for infusing culture into your life, but are they appropriate for your baby? Check with theater management to see if it's okay to hold your baby on your lap during the performance. The rules will vary from one venue to the next. Just make a mad dash for the door if the crying starts.

Trains: See airplane and bus, above.

Responding to Critics

Even when you're breastfeeding in a place and manner that seem
appropriate to you, you can't control how other people will react.
Everyone has an opinion, and there will definitely be a few people
who won't mind telling you theirs. Whether you're responding
to comments from family, friends, or complete strangers, rely on
psychology as you craft your reaction. There's no one-size-fits-all
response. Here are a couple common questions and a variety of
potential responses. Consider this your dress rehersal.

✿ *A relative asks, "So, how long are you planning
to breastfeed?"*

The polite answer: "I'm not entirely sure, but we'll
do whatever makes the most sense for the baby."

The flip answer: "Definitely before he goes to college."

The reverse-the-tables answer: "What would you recommend?"

The joke answer: "I'm not breastfeeding—these are
water balloons on my chest."

The mind-your-own-beeswax answer: "My husband
and I are planning to make the decision ourselves."

The real answer: "I don't know. Maybe when he turns
(insert age you plan to stop)."

From the Mouths of Moms

Breastfeeding used to be my ticket to cut lines. One time I started feeding Jake while waiting in a *long* line to get through security at an airport. Lo and behold, we were escorted to the front of the line.

— WENDY, OAKLAND, MAINE

❁ *A store employee says, "You're not allowed to do that here. I'm going to have to ask you to leave."*

The polite answer: "I'm sorry. I didn't think I was bothering anybody. I'll finish feeding and then continue shopping."

The flip answer: "Do what? I'm just shopping."

The reverse-the-tables answer: "Does anyone tell you where to eat lunch?"

The indignant answer: "Can I speak to the manager?"

The legal response: "This state has a law protecting my right to breastfeed here."

Chapter 6

HOW YOUR SPOUSE* CAN HELP

Whether your partner is a man or woman, and whether you're married or cohabitating, you're facing similar challenges. For simplicity's sake, this book uses the word "husband" or "spouse" to cover all situations.

Everyone tells you that having a baby can change the dynamic in your relationship. How can it not? You have a messy, noisy, and demanding new roommate. She'll start to cry just as you're about to "get it on" for the first time in months; she'll cry at 6 A.M., dashing your visions of a Sunday morning snuggled in bed; and she'll cry just as you're heading out the door for date night. Sounds romantic.

So here's the deal—you have to adapt. It's natural for there to be some tension as you go through this major life transition. But it doesn't have to descend into a bitter fight over whose turn it is to write thank-you notes, buy diapers, or clean the crud off the high chair. You aren't about to let your bundle of joy get the better of you, are you?

The key to preserving household harmony is sharing the load. It might be a cliché, but it's a cliché because it's based in truth. If one person is doing the lion's share of the baby "work," there's bound to be some resentment. The two of you can avoid any inequity by working out a good system for dividing and conquering.

Since most men can't lactate, that puts at least one task solidly in your court. But there's still a lot your spouse can do to help you. If he follows the Top Ten Breastfeeding Tips for Spouses, he'll be golden!

Top Ten Breastfeeding Tips for Spouses

(1) Provide words of encouragement and reassurance. Emotional support will make the new mom comfortable and confident about breastfeeding.

(2) Make sure the breastfeeding mother has all the supplies she needs for each feeding. Once she's stuck under the weight of a happily eating baby, it's not wise for her to get up and rock the boat. Things she might want: a glass of water, burp cloth, telephone, and television remote control.

(3) Think of a sweet way to surprise the breastfeeding mom. Flowers, a note, a foot rub, or perhaps a gift certificate for a spa will help her forget how tired she is.

(4) Give the baby a bottle of pumped breast milk or formula so that mom can nap or even sleep for four hours straight during the night. But before jumping in with that bottle, wait until a few weeks after birth so that mom's breastfeeding routine and milk supply are well established.

(5) Retrieve the baby when she cries in the middle of the night and take her to mom for a feeding. Once the feeding is over, burp and diaper the baby so that mom can go back to sleep.

(6) Help with housework. Babies generate a bottomless pile of dirty clothes, so do a load of laundry. In addition, do the dishes and clean some bottles.

(7) Take care of dinner at least a couple nights a week. If you aren't Emeril, then order take-out or pick up a pizza on your way home.

(8) Offer to write thank-you notes for baby gifts. At a minimum, make sure there are enough stamps in the house.

(9) Ask a breastfeeding mother, "Do you need help with anything while you're feeding the baby?" Even if she says "No," she'll definitely appreciate your concern.

(10) Photograph or videotape mom and baby while breastfeeding. Despite all protests, mom will probably be glad to have a photo to look back on.

Be Realistic

Nobody's perfect. It's idealistic to think that any spouse will be willing or able to follow all those tips. Sometimes your spouse will be right there, sorting through a week's worth of mail, recycling newspapers, *and* picking up his dirty gym clothes off the floor. Other times, he'll get sucked into his Blackberry and may not even hear your request to call the baby store to see if your new stroller has arrived. But he means well, so cut him some slack.

Besides, don't think you're home-free on all of this. You still have to do your share of work around the house. It's also your job to help your spouse help you. Let him take charge on certain things. Once he sees you trust him to give the baby a bath, he'll be more likely to offer to do so. And when he's elbow-deep in soapy water, try not to tell him which washcloth to use. If he's sensitive, your suggestions might hurt his feelings. Remember, there really are multiple ways to do this baby thing.

Finally, give your spouse time to bond with the baby. In the early days, some dads can feel left out of the breastfeeding party. For families who already have an older child, dad may have so much else to do around the house that he misses time with the newborn. So make a plan to get dad involved. He can always burp, diaper, and bathe the baby. He might even want to take off his shirt and lay the baby directly on his bare chest. Will the baby go for his nipple? Probably not. But if she

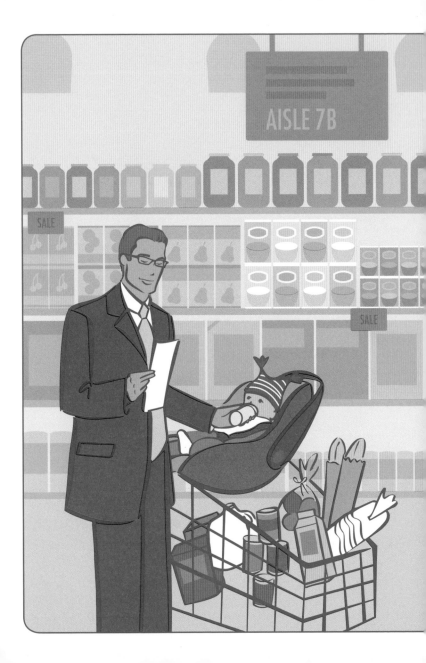

starts rooting around, bouncing her head against his chest and opening her mouth, at least you'll know what she's looking for. Then it's your turn to take over again. Just make sure he gets you a glass of water!

From the Mouths of Dads

Our son Azi was born a month early and hadn't yet developed his nursing instinct. Our midwife suggested that we feed him with a periodontal syringe. Holding Azi in my lap, I would put my pinky finger in his mouth and gently press it against his upper palate to get him to start sucking. I would then insert the curved tip of the syringe alongside my finger and dispense the breast milk my wife had pumped. As Azi grew stronger and learned to nurse, I still retained the privilege of our syringe feedings together. Sure, it meant that I would have to do a late-night feeding every once in a while, but it was worth it. Who says men can't breastfeed?

— CRAIG BORETH, SANTA MONICA, CALIFORNIA
Author of *How to Feel Manly in a Minivan*

Chapter 7

SEX AND RELAXATION

You're in bed. Your frisky husband is beside you. Your infant won't go to sleep. Do you (a) sing a lullabye to the baby; (b) get down to business with your husband; (c) pretend to be asleep; or (d) some combination of all of the above? If you answered (d), you're right there with the rest of us.

Being both a mom *and* a lover is often overwhelming and confusing. You're being pulled from all sides. Everyone wants a piece of you (*literally*), and all you want to do is sleep. Plus, now that your breasts are someone's main source of nutrition, it's sometimes hard to imagine they ever had another role. That silky black bra and thong you bought last year seem like ancient artifacts. Besides, you're fantasizing about sleep, not sex.

All women react differently to having a baby and breastfeeding. Some say their sex drive vanishes, whereas others find their libido as revved up as ever. Whatever your situation, try not to put too much pressure on yourself. It's going to take a while, months even, before you feel remotely like your old self. For starters, your doctor will probably tell you to abstain from sex and exercise for the first six weeks after giving birth. She'll want to make sure that everything "down there" has had enough time to heal properly.

This doctor's order may come as a relief for you—it's kind of hard to think about sex when you just squeezed a seven-pound bowling ball out from between your legs.

To get yourself back in the mood, you've got to take care of your body, your mind, and your relationship. It's like getting the oil changed in your car—it takes regular maintenance to keep the machinery running smoothly. Here are some tips for restoring body and soul.

For Your Body

✿ *Take a nap.* You may not sleep well for the next eighteen years, so do everything you can to give yourself a break.

✿ *Focus on nutrition.* Drink a lot of water and eat well-balanced meals. The weeks after giving birth are *not* the time to start dieting. You need sufficient calories and nutritious meals while you're breastfeeding.

✿ *Shave your legs.* Just think, for the first time in months you can actually reach your legs without bumping into your stomach!

✿ *Get your hair cut and colored.* You may *feel* seventy-five years old, but you don't have to look it.

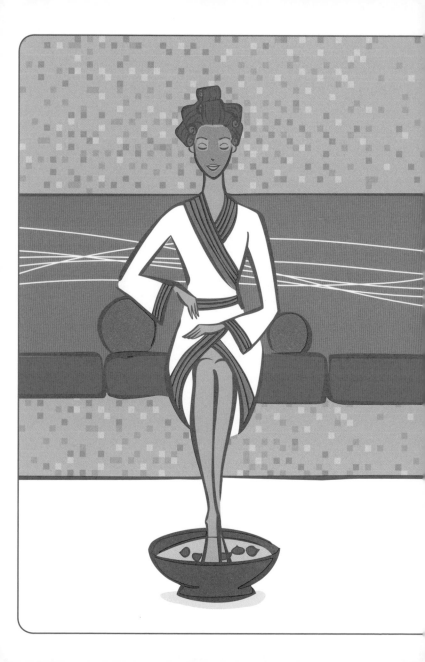

❀ *Get a massage.* Your arms may start to ache from holding your baby all the time, so a professional massage can do wonders. If you don't want to spend the money, ask your spouse to do the honors.

❀ *Get a facial.* If you don't have the cash, buy a mask to do at home. Close the bathroom door and tell everyone to leave you alone for half an hour.

❀ *Get a pedicure.* Washing your hands twenty thousand times a day will ruin a manicure, so treat your toes instead.

❀ *Get some exercise.* Take the baby for a walk. The fresh air is good for both of you. Plus, pushing fifty pounds of baby, stroller, and gear is a good workout. Once you get the go-ahead from your doctor, embrace your inner jock.

❀ *Do Kegel exercises.* Kegels are helpful to restore muscle tone to your vagina and pelvic floor. Sit on the floor or in a chair with your knees bent, then clench and release the muscles of your vagina. Do these ten times, at least once a day. (Everyone knows they should do these exercises, but few people seem to have the discipline. Try to be the exception.)

❀ *Try a solo run.* If you're worried that sex will hurt, you can always test things out on your own. Masturbation might reassure you that your machinery still works.

For Your Brain

✿ **Read.** Parenting books *do not* count. Read a book or magazine that has absolutely nothing to do with babies.

✿ **Go to the movies with your baby.** Check local theaters to see if they offer special screening times for moms and newborns. This will be one showing where you won't have to whisper.

✿ **Catch up on your favorite TV shows.** Hours spent breastfeeding on the couch are the perfect time to watch television. A digital video recorder will record your favorite shows with minimal effort on your part; you'll never have to watch a commercial again!

✿ **Hang out with an old friend.** If you can't get someone to watch the baby, bring him along. He'll probably sleep. If not, feed him, and he'll doze off.

✿ **Make new friends.** Find a group for new parents at your local community center. You may be relieved to hear others share their stories about the wild, wild West of parenthood.

✿ **Spread your news.** Call or e-mail people to tell them about the new addition to your family.

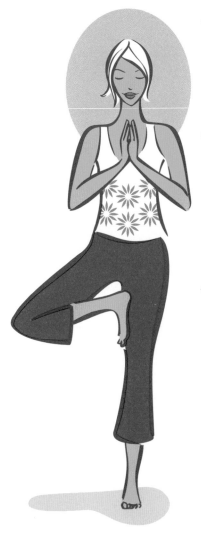

❀ *Practice yoga.* Yoga encourages the type of breathing that can help you control anxiety and clear your head.

❀ *Meditate.* Meditation is a proven relaxation method, but it's not easy to achieve the Zen state of a Buddhist monk. Find a class, book, or Web site to guide you through the process.

❀ *Reconnect to the office— but only if you want to.* You may or may not want to check in with your colleagues. For some, checking e-mail and voicemail might be a good break from taking care of the baby. For others, work just leads to stress. If that sounds like you, then take advantage of your maternity leave and *don't do any work.*

Mama Data

The ancient Greeks credited the creation of the Milky Way to a breast-feeding mishap. Zeus apparently gave his illegitimate son Hercules to his wife, Hera, to breastfeed. When Hera realized Hercules was not her son, she pushed him away and her milk sprayed into the heavens, creating the Milky Way, that luminous band of stars that spreads across the sky.

✿ *Hire someone to help.* If family members aren't available to lend a hand, and you have enough money to hire help, an extra body can seem like a savior. A night-nurse can take care of the baby overnight. A postpartum doula can take care of the baby and do some cooking and cleaning during the day. Then there are always the traditional housekeepers, baby sitters, and nannies. But before you hire someone, thoroughly check references.

For Your Relationship

✿ ***Recognize that your spouse is adjusting, too.*** You may
be the one who had the baby, but he's sort of postpartum, too.
Some guys can feel overwhelmed by their new sense of
responsibility. So be mindful of his feelings. Do something
to make sure he knows how much you appreciate his help.
A simple "thank you" is a good place to start.

✿ ***Romance your spouse.*** Remember the time in your life
when dating was a series of fun surprises and activities that
you plotted and planned? Well, it's time to try all that again.
At a minimum, sending a flirtatious e-mail will give you
something different to think about while you're caught in
the daily poop-feed-poop-feed cycle.

✿ ***Talk, talk, talk.*** Make sure you're still communicating about
things other than the baby and household responsibilities.

✿ ***Train a sitter.*** Teach her how you change a diaper, give
a bottle, and put the baby to sleep. Before long, you can leave
her alone with the baby so that you and your husband can
get away for a while. Just make an emergency contact list
and post it on the refrigerator door before you go.

❀ **Go on a date.** If your baby isn't taking a bottle, you may not be able to leave for very long—but even two hours out of the house will be a nice break for the two of you.

❀ **Have date night in your own home.** If you don't want to leave the baby alone with the sitter yet, the two of you can hide out in your bedroom. Tell the sitter to come get you only in an emergency.

❀ **Spend a night in a hotel.** Once you feel comfortable with your sitter and you've established a solid breastfeeding routine, book a night at a hotel. You don't even have to leave town to feel like you've escaped. Just be sure to leave behind enough pumped milk or formula to get the baby through the night. Don't forget to pack your pump!

❀ **Take it slow.** It will be a little while before things feel totally back to normal, but once you two are alone, you'll know just what to do. After all, that's how you got into this situation in the first place. If you're really having a hard time getting in the mood, try some erotica or one of those premium cable TV channels.

And cut your breasts some slack. Once you do get things going, your breasts might feel a little different than they did before you had your baby. They may feel tender or desensitized to stimulation. They may also leak or even spray milk during sex! That's because breastfeeding and orgasms involve the release of the same hormone, oxytocin.

✿ *Schedule sex.* This doesn't sound too romantic, but it can make a difference. Figure out what time of day works the best for the two of you. Too tired at night? Make a plan for the morning. No time in the morning? Schedule a rendezvous during the baby's nap. Or how about this—ask your spouse if he'd like to "E.F. or F.F?" In other words, does he want to "Eat First or F**k First?" Dinner before play, or play before dinner? And by all means, USE A LUBRICANT DURING SEX! Pregnancy and breastfeeding hormones can make your vagina dry. Get out that KY.

✿ *See a couples therapist if you need to.* Exhaustion and new responsibilities are sometimes a toxic mix. It's common to fight. But if things are really overwhelming, seek help. Find a third party, a trusted relative or friend, or even a therapist to advise you. Don't allow yourself to take drastic steps while you're still adjusting to your new roommate.

Chapter 8

WEANING YOUR BABY
. . . AND YOURSELF

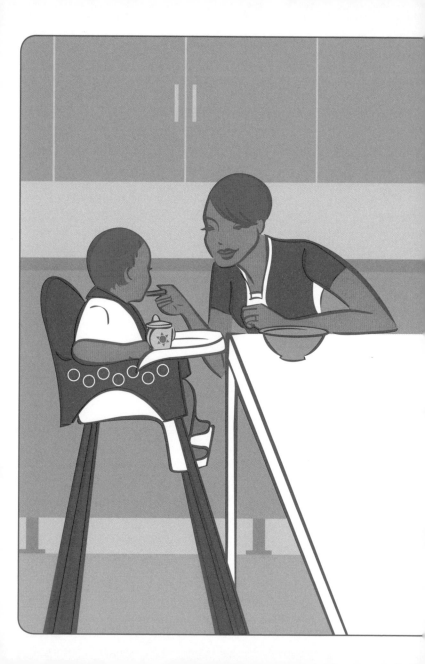

At some point, it will be time to stop breastfeeding.
For some, the moment comes a few days after birth.
For others, it's weeks, months, or a year later. Some
truly committed breastfeeders will even stick with
it for a couple years or more.

Like all parenting decisions, weaning can be
fraught with emotions. It's impossible not to wonder
if you're making the right decision about your timing.
So don't be surprised if you get a little weepy as your
nursing relationship draws to a close. Sometimes,
moms even feel depressed during this transition
since weaning can trigger hormonal changes. If you
are unusually sad, talk to someone about how you
feel. And remember—even though you won't have
the same extended cuddling sessions, you'll always
have memories of the special bond you and your baby
formed. Weaning is just one of the many separations
you'll face as a parent. Today it's weaning; before you
know it, it's high-school graduation. After all, that's
what we signed up for.

When to Wean

There isn't a strict rule about when to wean your baby. Some moms initiate weaning, guiding the baby through the process. Others let the baby take charge and wean at her own pace, usually well into toddlerhood. Basically, it's a personal choice. You have to do what works best for you, your baby, and your family.

In the United States, most medical professionals encourage moms to breastfeed as long as they are willing to do so. The American Academy of Pediatrics (AAP) recommends that moms give infants *only breast milk* for the first six months after the baby is born. That means no formula, water, juice, or solid foods. The AAP also suggests that mothers breastfeed (in addition to feeding the baby solid foods) until the baby is at least one year old. Other organizations, such as the World Health Organization (WHO), recommend breastfeeding, in addition to feeding solids, for two years.

If you decide to wean before the baby is one year old, you will need to give her bottles of pumped breast milk or formula until her first birthday. Once she's a year old, she can have cow's milk. By the age of one, some doctors recommend that the baby use a sippy cup rather than a bottle.

From the Mouths of Moms

Even before I got pregnant, I had it all planned out. My child would breastfeed until he bit me and never use a pacifier, watch TV, or eat fast-food. Ahem. I tried to keep up with my plan, but when my son's first teeth appeared, neither one of us was ready to stop nursing. So I told people—almost apologetically—that we would stop when he turned one year old. Well, he turned one, and again, neither of us was ready to end it. That's when I started joking—"When he can ask for his preferred breast, *that's* when we'll stop." Well, my son nursed until he was three—well beyond that stage, too. I'm happily breastfeeding my new baby daughter now, and we'll nurse as long as she likes. In fact, it's time to nurse right now. As soon as I put down this chicken nugget, I'll take the pacifier out of her mouth, turn off Zoboomafoo, and we'll get started. No false deadlines—or preconceived notions—this time around.

— KARI ANNE ROY, AUSTIN, TEXAS
Author of *Haiku Mama*

How to Wean

Most babies won't be ready to call it quits exactly when you are. In fact, some experts say that if it was up to the baby, weaning wouldn't start until well after age one and might not even happen until the child is between two and four years old. If your baby seems like she's trying to wean but she's still pretty young, she may actually be on "strike." This is a temporary setback rather than true self-weaning. Possible causes include household stress (moving, a family crisis), illness, teething, and new perfume or soap. If you think an external circumstance is affecting your baby, remedy the situation, provide as much cuddling as possible, and try to continue nursing.

If you're ready for a change but your baby isn't, how do you encourage her to give up her most prized possession in the entire universe? Here are some guidelines.

✿ ***Don't quit cold turkey.*** Even if you're really ready to wean, don't just stop without warning. Definitely don't wean by deserting your baby for a weekend away. Your baby will be miserable and you'll be pretty uncomfortable, too, since you'll still have a supply of milk.

❧ ***Drop one feeding at a time.*** Shorten, and then eliminate, one feeding at a time. Substitute either a bottle or a sippy cup in place of your breast. Spend a week, or at least a few days, with your new feeding schedule. Once you and the baby are comfortable, cut back another feeding.

❧ ***Follow the "don't offer, don't refuse" principle.*** Only breastfeed your baby when she asks for it. Don't encourage her to eat if she's not really hungry.

❧ ***Distraction, distraction, distraction.*** When your baby wants to nurse, give him a favorite toy, take a walk, snuggle, or visit friends.

❧ ***Change your feeding routines.*** If you always sit in the same chair to nurse, stop using that chair.

❧ ***Change the sleeping arrangements.*** If the baby is sleeping with you, think about other options. Have her sleep next to dad, move her to her own crib, or move her crib to another room.

❧ ***Get others to help.*** If your baby always nurses first thing in the morning when you pick her up, send your spouse in to do the morning routine. He can give her a bottle or a sippy cup of milk.

❀ ***Continue to snuggle.*** Make sure your baby gets plenty of additional cuddling time as you're weaning. The physical contact is reassuring to her. Odds are you'll want a good snuggle, too.

❀ ***Pump to relieve pressure.*** If you find yourself getting engorged between feedings, use a breast pump to express just enough milk so that you're no longer engorged. Don't pump too much, or you'll continue to stimulate milk production. Be on the lookout for signs of engorgement or mastitis.

❀ ***Consider partial weaning.*** It's not necessary to wean entirely. In fact, some moms will give up all but one or two feedings.

❀ ***Talk to your doctor before initiating sudden weaning.*** In some instances, a medical condition, or the need for surgery, may cause some moms to consider weaning quickly. Before doing so, seek multiple medical opinions and do your homework to learn about your individual condition.

❀ ***Don't bind your breasts.*** You might hear that some women bind their breasts (wrap them tightly) during weaning. This practice isn't proven to reduce pain or swelling and is therefore not recommended. Wearing a supportive bra is enough.

❧ ***Let her pick a day to stop.*** If you're weaning a toddler,
you may be able to talk to her about the change and let her
play an active role in it. You might even consider having
a "weaning party" to celebrate her reaching her milestone.
(Or should we say *your* milestone?)

❧ ***Be patient.*** Don't expect weaning to end on a specific day.
It could take weeks, or even months, but you'll be packing
away your nursing bras before you know it.

From the Mouths of Moms

I nursed Kiki for twenty-three months and was concerned it would
be hard to wean her. My pediatrician suggested I try a unique ap-
proach—putting Band-Aids over my nipples and telling her my boobies
were "broken." Kiki would say, "Mama, pick me up—I want boobies."
I would tell her they were broken, and lift my shirt to show her the
Band-Aids. She would curiously examine them, look at me sadly,
and say, "Oh shame, Mama. So sorry about it. Boobies are broken."
This went on for a week. But the best part—as soon as she was weaned,
she slept through the night for the first time in her life.

— LEANNE, JOHANNESBURG, SOUTH AFRICA

A Final Thought—Weaning Mom

Nothing ever turns out exactly as you think it will.
"I don't think I'll be able to breastfeed," you might say.
But then your baby nurses like an old pro. "My baby
will never have an ounce of formula," you might decide.
But then you end up supplementing.

The same goes for weaning. You'll set an end date.
Then, lo and behold, it changes. You push it back because
your baby is sick. You move it up because you have
a business trip. Your goals change from day to day.

So wean yourself. Wean yourself of all your
preconceived notions about breastfeeding. It might be
tough. It may even be as challenging as weaning your
baby from nursing. But there's a reward to letting go of
your opinions and concerns—when things take a different
course than you envision, it's easier to go with the flow.

In some ways, that's the beauty of this whole
Mama thing. You get to make it up as you go along.
No matter what anyone else says—and they'll be sure
to say a lot—you're the one who decides how to feed
your baby. You're the Mama, and Mama Knows Breast.

Resources

Instructional Books

Eiger, Marvin S., M.D., and Sally Wendkos Olds. *The Complete Book of Breastfeeding.* (Bantam Books, 1999)

Hale, Thomas W., Ph.D. *Medications and Mothers' Milk.* (Hale Publishing, L.P., 2006)

Huggins, Kathleen, R.N., M.S. *The Nursing Mother's Companion.* (Harvard Common Press, 2005)

La Leche League International. *The Womanly Art of Breastfeeding.* (Plume, 2004)

Newman, Jack, M.D., and Teresa Pitman. *The Ultimate Breastfeeding Book of Answers.* (Three Rivers Press, 2006)

Sears, Martha, R.N., and William Sears, M.D. *The Breastfeeding Book.* (Little, Brown and Company, 2000)

Tamaro, Janet. *So That's What They're For! Breastfeeding Basics.* (Adams Media, 1998)

Mom to Mom Books

Behrmann, Barbara L. *The Breastfeeding Café: Mothers Share the Joys, Challenges, & Secrets of Nursing.* (University of Michigan Press, 2005)

Colburn-Smith, Cate, and Andrea Serrette. *The Milk Memos: How*

Real Moms Learned to Mix Business with Babies–and How You Can, Too. (Tarcher Penguin, 2007)

Giles, Fiona. *Fresh Milk: The Secret Life of Breasts.* (Simon & Schuster, 2003)

Steiner, Andy. *Spilled Milk: Breastfeeding Adventures and Advice from Less-Than-Perfect Moms.* (Rodale, 2005)

Web Sites

www.aap.org (The American Academy of Pediatrics): Covers everything from ear infections to car seat safety, including comprehensive breastfeeding information.

www.askdrsears.com: Advice from pediatrician guru Dr. Sears.

www.bfar.org (Breastfeeding After Breast and Nipple Surgeries): Information about breastfeeding after all types of breast surgery, especially implants and reductions.

www.bflrc.info (Bright Future Lactation Resource Centre, Ltd.): Information from well-known lactation consultant Linda Smith, IBCLC.

www.breastfeeding.com: Wide range of information for moms.

www.checkyourboobies.org (Check Your Boobies): Official site of an organization run by a woman who developed breast cancer while breastfeeding. Sign up for a monthly e-mail reminding you to do a breast self-exam.

http://community.lsoft.com/archives/LACTNET.html (LactNet): Lactation professionals frequent this discussion group, but anyone can join.

www.kathydettwyler.org: Official site of Dr. Katherine Dettwyler; offers an anthropologist's take on breastfeeding issues.

www.drjacknewman.com: Dr. Jack Newman's official site; offers expert breastfeeding advice and information.

www.hmbana.org: (Human Milk Banking Association of North America): Information about donating breast milk.

www.ilca.org: (International Lactation Consultant Association): Use this site to find a lactation consultant.

www.iblce.org: (International Board of Lactation Consultant Examiners): A site for professional lactation consultants, with interesting information for moms, too.

www.kellymom.com: Breastfeeding and parenting site with informative articles and a good chat room for moms.

www.lalecheleague.org: The official site for La Leche League; easy to search for specific information.

www.mamaknowsbreast.com: The place to go for the latest breastfeeding news, tips, and anecdotes.

www.ncsl.org (National Conference of State Legislatures): To find out the breastfeeding law in your state, type "breastfeeding" into the search bar.

www.promom.org (Promotion of Mother's Milk, Inc.): This site has good breastfeeding information and discussion groups.

www.toxnet.nlm.nih.gov (TOXNET). The U.S. National Library of Medicine runs this site, which offers information on the safety of individual medications while breastfeeding. Click on LactMed.

www.waba.org.my (World Alliance for Breastfeeding Action): Promotes breastfeeding worldwide.

Index

Acknowledgments

I could not have written this book without *a lot* of help.
I'd like to thank pediatricians Dr. Stephanie Freilich
and Dr. Harold Raucher; Ob-Gyn Dr. Dawn Kopel;
the numerous lactation consultants, including Andrea
Syms-Brown, IBCLC, RLC, CIMI, who reviewed the
book and provided wise counsel; my husband, Scott,
who encouraged me to keep at it, especially when
the book deal and our second son were born the same
week; my sons, who gave me plenty of time to ponder
the vagaries of breastfeeding; my ultimate cheerleaders,
my nuclear family; Toby Schmidt, who gave me the
idea to write this book; my babysitters Sara Heinze,
Rebecca Schumer, and Vilma Taraskeviciute; my agent,
Katherine Fausset, whose sense of humor helped me
hone my book proposal; and, of course, Melissa Wagner,
my editor at Quirk Books.

About the Author

Andi Silverman was first inspired to breastfeed by her mom. While her mom nursed her brother, Andi occupied herself with a doll and toy diaper bag, though she ran into problems actually "feeding" her doll.

Thirty-plus years later, Andi learned the true art of breast-feeding with back-to-back pregnancies. Her sons, who are eighteen months apart, taught her the fundamentals of the "milky way."

Prior to breastfeeding for hours on end, Andi was a lawyer and a television reporter. She reported for the CBS and Fox affiliates in Boston and an NBC station in Charlottesville, Virginia. She is also the founder of Scoop Productions (www. scoopproductions.com), a video production company. She is a graduate of Brown University, the University of Virginia School of Law, and the Columbia University Graduate School of Journalism.

Andi also runs the blog www.mamaknowsbreast.com.

About the Illustrator

Cindy Luu graduated from Rhode Island School of Design and quickly found herself designing for both Estée Lauder and Bloomingdales. She has illustrated many books and has her own line of greeting cards. This book was of particular importance to her, as her two-year-old son Matthew was by her side for the entire process.